PROTECT
YOUR FAMILY!

PROTECT
YOUR FAMILY!

Don't Write a Blank Check
to the Nursing Home

WE'VE CRACKED THE CODE ON
LONG-TERM CARE PLANNING

Advantage®

Published by Advantage, Charleston, South Carolina.
Member of Advantage Media Group.

ADVANTAGE is a registered trademark and the Advantage colophon is a trademark of Advantage Media Group, Inc.

Printed in the United States of America.

ISBN: 978-159932-665-8
LCCN: 2012930889

Advantage Media Group is proud to be a part of the Tree Neutral® program. Tree Neutral offsets the number of trees consumed in the production and printing of this book by taking proactive steps such as planting trees in direct proportion to the number of trees used to print books. To learn more about Tree Neutral, please visit www.treeneutral.com. To learn more about Advantage's commitment to being a responsible steward of the environment, please visit www.advantagefamily.com/green

Advantage Media Group is a leading publisher of business, motivation, and self-help authors. Do you have a manuscript or book idea that you would like to have considered for publication? Please visit www.amgbook.com or call 1.866.775.1696

DISCLAIMER

This book does not constitute and should not be treated as legal advice. The authors do not assume responsibility for your reliance on or use of the information in this book. You should contact an elder law attorney for advice regarding your particular circumstances. Furthermore, the authors do not assume responsibility for any errors or omissions in this book. Although every effort has been made to assure the accuracy of the information in this book at the time of the writing of this book, laws and regulations are constantly changing. You should contact an elder law attorney before taking any action with regard to your estate and long-term health care planning.

FOREWORD

"A SOCIETY GROWS GREAT WHEN
OLD MEN AND WOMEN PLANT TREES
WHOSE SHADE THEY KNOW THEY
SHALL NEVER SIT IN."

– Greek proverb

Throughout history, smart people have recognized the wisdom of their elders and the value of getting good advice.

In the cradle of democracy, the ancient Greeks formed their councils to take advantage of the collective wisdom of the smartest – i.e. oldest – people in their society. Centuries later, it was the Roman Senate that held great power. Indeed, the word "Senate" comes from the Latin *senex*, which means "the council of elders."

Our own American experience reflects similar reverence for the wisdom gathered by leaders over a lifetime. Even as young men and women were driving the American Revolution, they turned to elder statesmen like Ben Franklin for guidance. Indeed, it was Franklin who advocated a model of government – in some ways based upon the ancient Greek and Roman concepts, but also on the Iroquois Native American model – which encouraged respect for age.

We all recognize the value of having a mentor, a trusted advisor we can go to for answers to our most difficult questions. For some of us, that's our spouse or our grandparent or a trusted friend. The problem is, when it comes to legal issues or caregiving advice, we're not likely to have anyone in our circle who truly knows the answers to our most heartfelt concerns. So we just carry on, resigned to doing the best we can, knowing that we are probably missing opportunities or not taking the steps we ought to be taking . . . but not even knowing where to begin or who to turn to.

I recently received an email from Julie Steinbacher telling me about the "Dream Team" of elder law attorneys she had assembled to write a book on long-term care planning. I am a practicing elder law attorney as well, and Julie wanted to get my feedback on the manuscript. I told her I'd be happy to take a look at it, but in the back of my mind, I've got to admit I wasn't all that excited about reading a book about an area of the law where I'd been practicing for the last fifteen years.

I received a copy of the manuscript, and I glanced at it a few days before my wife and I were to go on vacation. As I started reading, I immediately realized that this book was very different. The co-authors are all leaders in the elder law field – but much more than that, they all have an ability to communicate difficult material in a way the layperson can understand.

I brought the book along with me on vacation (much to the chagrin of my wife, Mary) and the more I read, the more excited I became. That's when I realized that this book reminded me of the ancient Greek and Roman councils I mentioned earlier. This truly is a work put together by the brightest in the field, each writing in his or her particular area of interest. As soon as I finished the manuscript, I emailed Julie and asked her if I could write the foreword. I wanted to have my name associated with this wonderful book, at least in some small way.

Can you imagine sitting down in your living room with some of the brightest stars in the elder law field and being able to pick their brains for less than the cost of a night at the movies? Here's just a tiny bit of what you might learn:

- How can I get help paying for the cost of long-term care?
- How can I qualify for benefits from the VA?
- Who needs a will and who doesn't?
- Who should have a power of attorney and why?
- What is a reverse mortgage and when does it make sense?
- How do I deal with end-of-life concerns?
- What housing options should I be looking at?
- When should I prepare for getting older?
  (Hint: It wasn't raining when Noah built the ark.)
- What tips do the best caregivers use to take care of their loved ones and themselves?
- . . . and so much more.

As I'm writing this foreword, I've got to admit I'm struggling. But they say confession is good for the soul, so I'll come right out and say it.

THIS IS THE BOOK I WISH I HAD WRITTEN.

Unfortunately, even after fifteen years of practicing elder law on a daily basis, I simply don't have the collective wisdom that this group of elder law attorneys has. The fact that you're reading this book means that you have an opportunity to take care of yourself and your family in a way few others will ever understand. I truly believe this is a life-changing book for those fortunate enough to read it and act upon it. The attorneys who have taken time to write this book have given you and me a great gift. Read this book and follow the advice given. This is the path to peace of mind. And, after all, isn't that what each of us wants?

The anthropologist, Margaret Meade, once said, "Never doubt that a small group of thoughtful, committed citizens can change the world – indeed, it is the only thing that ever has."

I now understand what she was talking about.

William G. Hammond, JD
www.kcelderlaw.com

TABLE OF CONTENTS

CHAPTER 1

HOW TO PREPARE
FOR GETTING OLDER

Michelle D. Beneski, LLM in Taxation,
CELA

Certified Elder Law Attorney by the
National Elder Law Foundation

Accredited Attorney by the Veterans Administration

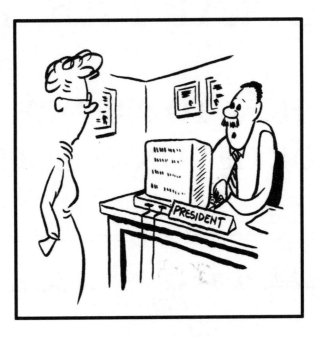

"MRS. HIGGINS, WHICH BUTTON
DO I PUSH TO MAKE A
SMILEY FACE."

"IT WASN'T RAINING WHEN NOAH BUILT THE ARK."

– Howard J. Ruff (1931 to -)
Financial Adviser and Writer

"FAILURE TO PREPARE IS PREPARING TO FAIL."

– John Wooden (1910-2010)
Basketball Player and Basketball Coach

§ 1.4.   Do You Want to Protect Assets From the Cost of Long-Term Care?

§ 1.4.1.   The Cost of Long-Term Care

§ 1.4.2.   How Are You Going to Pay for Long-Term Care?

§ 1.5.   A Long-Term Care Plan

§ 1.5.1.   What is a Long-Term Care Plan?

Not many people like to contemplate getting older. Because we do not like to think about it, we often do not prepare for our old age. It sneaks up on is before we know it. There are certain areas of our life about which we should consider and plan. Here are some questions to think about:

- Where will you live if you can not take care of yourself?
- Who will make your medical decisions if you cannot make them for yourself?
- Does that person know your wishes for medical care?
- Who will manage your finances if you cannot manage them yourself?
- How will the person who is managing your finances get access to your assets?
- Do you want to preserve assets for future generations or do you want to spend as much as needed to pay for your care?
- How are you going to pay for any long-term care that you may need?
- How much do you think your long-term care needs will cost?
- Do you know what government benefits you may need and how to qualify for them?

I'm sure there are more questions that should be answered but this is a good start. The purpose of this chapter is not to answer all of these questions but rather to raise issues to consider. Other chapters in this book will cover certain topics in more detail.

§ 1.1.
WHERE WILL YOU LIVE IF YOU CANNOT TAKE CARE OF YOURSELF?

§ 1.1.1. Living at Home

When I ask this question of clients the usual answer is "I'm going to stay in my home until I die." This is possible but if you are truly going to live at home, you have to consider how you will be cared for at home, how the care be paid for, and who will do the caregiving. If you do not answer these questions, you probably will not be able to stay at home until your death.

Is your home set up for someone in a wheel chair or someone who cannot climb stairs? If not, find out how much it will cost to renovate in case you need to renovate. How will you pay for this renovation? Do you have enough savings or perhaps you are thinking about a reverse mortgage?

If you cannot live alone, who will live with you to care for you? Will a child move in? Have you discussed this with the child and just as importantly have you discussed it with all your other children (if any)? I have seen many families torn apart because one child moves in to take care of a parent but another child in the family does not agree with how the parent is being cared for in the home. Your wish to stay at home should be covered in your living will. See the chapter of this book on powers of attorney and living wills. Will you hire caregivers? Should you pay family members to care for you? How do you expect to pay for this care? Medicaid, Veteran's benefits, savings, long-term care insurance, and a reverse mortgage are all possible options. Read the chapters on these topics to see if your expectation is realistic and whether you need to do anything to prepare. Let your family know you have a plan by writing it down. It is perfectly okay to decide that you want to spend every penny you have to stay at home even if your entire estate is depleted. However, if the person managing your health care decisions and your finances does not know your wish, he or she may decide that some other living arrangement is better for either health or financial reasons.

Your best chance of staying at home for as long as possible is directly tied to the planning you do now to prepare for the future. The ostrich's head in the sand approach to avoiding issues will not work here.

§ 1.1.2. Living Some Place Other Than Home

There are many options for seniors who cannot live at home. Some options to consider include an independent apartment in a complex that supplies extra support when needed, senior housing, an assisted living facility, a child's or friend's home, a rest home, or a nursing home. There is a whole chapter on housing options. Please read it. Just as with living at home, you need to ask yourself: how will you be cared for, how will the care be paid, and who will do the caregiving. Your plan should include when you think it is appropriate for you to be moved out of your home if you are not capable of communicating your wishes and your preference as to where you would like to live if you cannot live at home.

§ 1.2.
PLANNING FOR HEALTH CARE DECISIONS

§ 1.2.1. Who Will Make Your Medical Decisions for You if You Cannot Make Them for Yourself?

We would all like to live a long and healthy life. However, the lifetime chance of a person over age 65 developing a disability that lasts at least three months affecting at least two activities of daily living[1] or becoming cognitively impaired is 44% for men and 72% for women.[2] The risk should not be ignored.

If you should become disabled and cannot make your own medical decisions and have not executed a document authorizing someone to make medical decisions for you, then the court will appoint someone to make your medical decisions. The court may not appoint the person you would have selected. This process is known as a guardianship. In many states the fact that you are related to a person does not automatically entitle the relative to make medical decisions for you.

You can avoid the need for a guardianship in most situations by executing a health care power of attorney.[3] We have included a whole chapter on powers of attorney. Please read that chapter carefully.

When considering who you should pick to be your health care agent consider the following:

- Who will follow your wishes rather than his or her own wishes?
- Who has a good understanding of medical issues?
- Who has the emotional fortitude to make difficult decisions?

Please do not pick "the oldest" or even "the nurse or doctor" if you do not believe that person will be able to do what you want them to do.

§ 1.2.2. Does Your Health Care Agent Understand What You Would Want Done or Not Done for Your Health Care?

Making life and death decisions for another person is a tremendous burden. You may believe that the person knows, but are you sure? If you picked your spouse as your health care agent and your child as an alternate, does your child know? It is best to write down for your agent what medical procedures you want or do not want and how you want to be cared for. In some states this is known as a "living will" or "advanced health care directive." In some states a living will is legally binding on the agent. The agent cannot act in a manner inconsistent with the living will. In other states, the living will is merely a statement of your wishes or intent. In those states the health care agent can make what ever decision the health care agent deems best and the living will is provided as guidance.

Even if your health care agent knows your wishes and the state does not consider the living will legally binding, you should still execute a living will document. Why? Because it may give the health care agent some piece of mind. It also may resolve any family conflict over what type of care you would or would not want. It may also be useful to the health care agent in any discussions with doctors who want to provide or not provide a certain medical procedure. Please read the chapter on powers of attorney/health care directives and the chapter on end of life issues. Both should be helpful in choosing a health care agent and letting that agent know what type of care you want or do not want.

§ 1.3.
PLANNING FOR FINANCIAL DECISIONS

§ 1.3.1. Who Will Manage Your Finances if You Cannot Manage Them Yourself?

Similar to health care decisions, if you should become disabled and cannot manage your finances and have not executed a document authorizing someone to manage your finances for you, then the court will appoint someone to manage your finances The court may not appoint the person you would have selected. This process is known in some states as a conservatorship and in others as a guardianship.

Many clients tell me that they do not need a power of attorney because "all our accounts are joint." Clients are surprised to find out that a spouse cannot take money out of your Individual Retirement Account (IRA) even if it is needed for your care and your spouse is the beneficiary on of the account. Your spouse or child cannot change the deed for your house or the ownership of your life insurance.

Joint accounts may be convenient for paying bills but joint accounts cannot authorize a person to other activities that may be necessary to take care of you in the future. Joint accounts are not enough!! You can avoid the need for a conservatorship or a guardianship in most situations by executing a financial durable power of attorney. We have included a whole chapter on powers of attorney. Please read that chapter carefully.

When considering who you should pick to be your agent, consider the following:

- Do not pick a person who is going through a divorce.
- Do not pick a person with financial problems.
- Do not pick a person who is not honest.
- Select someone you trust.
- Select someone you have known a long time.
- Select someone who manages his own finances well and is financially stable.

§ 1.3.2. How Will the Person Who Is Managing Your Finances Get Access to Your Assets?

Your agent under your power of attorney can access your bank accounts, your retirement accounts, and your life insurance policies. Your agent can also change the deed to your home and change the beneficiary of your life insurance policies. A power of attorney is one device for your agent to use in managing your assets.

Another device is a revocable or irrevocable trust. A trust is a written document that defines how the property within the trust is used. The person who administers the property in the trust according to the terms of the trust is known as the trustee. A trustee can only manage property that is owned by the trust. Usually with a revocable living trust, you are the trustee of your trust. However if you become ill and cannot act as trustee, you will usually have named someone else to be the successor trustee. A successor trustee steps into the role of trustee when the current trustee cannot act. This book contains a chapter on trusts (revocable and irrevocable) that you should review. Even if you have a trust, you should also have a power of attorney because a trustee has no authority to act regarding property outside of the trust. An agent under a power of attorney can act with regard to property outside the trust but not property within the trust. These documents work together.

§ 1.4.
DO YOU WANT TO PROTECT ASSETS FROM THE COST OF LONG-TERM CARE?

§ 1.4.1. The Cost of Long-Term Care

Long-term care costs could be home care costs, assisted living care costs, or nursing home costs. These costs can be substantial. These costs can deplete a family's savings in a very short period of time. Some clients come to us to request assistance in sheltering assets so that the assets do not have to be spent on the clients' care. Sometimes assets can be protected from the cost of care depending on, among other factors, your assets, your family, your state, and your illness.

The first question to ask yourself is "Do you want to protect your assets from the costs of long-term care and, if so, why?" I have many clients who desire to remain at home as long as possible and hopefully never enter a skilled nursing facility. If there is not an important reason to protect assets for children or other beneficiaries then it makes sense to use those assets to stay at home even if it depletes the estate.

There are reasons a person might want to pay privately for care. Perhaps the client desires a private room at the nursing home. Private rooms are often only available to those residents who privately pay for care. In some states assisted living facilities must be paid for privately. Quality of life is often better at an assisted living facility than a nursing home, and, therefore, clients who cannot manage at home may want to live in the assisted living. Many times the government benefits available to pay for home care are not really sufficient to keep a person at home. If the client wants to stay at home then either the person's family must supply care or caregivers must be hired privately.

Clients often come to an elder law attorney asking for help in protecting the family home and sometimes other assets from the cost of care so that the assets can be given to children or other heirs. I hear all the time "I worked my whole life for this house, and I don't want the government to get it; it's the only thing I have to give to my children." There are ways to protect the home and other assets from having to be sold to pay for care but these methods can be complicated. In several chapters of this book we discuss qualifying for Veterans benefits, Medicaid, subsidized housing, long-term care insurance, and reverse mortgages. Each of these topics can be used in the appropriate circumstance as a tool to protect assets from the cost of care. These chapters should be reviewed to determine which if any of these programs are suitable in your situation.

§ 1.4.2. How Are You Going to Pay for Long-Term Care?

In order to know how you are going to pay for care, you really need to know how much long-term care costs in your area. The cost varies significantly from place to place. In Massachusetts, the average cost of a nursing home is over $10,000 a month, assisted living costs start at around $5,000 a month, and private home care starts at about $20 an hour. All of these figures change regularly so please do not rely on them. Rather, find out what the current cost of care is in your town. Call some nursing homes, assisted livings, and home care agencies and ask for the daily or monthly rate. Once you know what care costs, then you need to consider how you will pay for the care you desire or need.

We have discussed earlier that private paying for care is an option. Private payment is often expensive and can deplete a person's savings quickly. There are several other methods available to pay for long-term care. Long-term care insurance is insurance that pays for care at home, in an assisted living facility, or in a nursing home. Medicaid can pay for care both at home and in a nursing home if you qualify for the program. Medicaid must be applied for, and the applicant must meet strict income and asset limits. Veteran's benefits are available to certain war-time veterans and certain disabled veterans to pay for care. Medicare pays for a limited amount of rehabilitation care at home or in a nursing home. There is a chapter on each one of these topics in this book. Please explore which if any of these programs you might be able to qualify for.

It is important to plan for care before you need it. Once you are aware of how much care costs and the type of care you want or need, then you need to work with an elder law attorney to prepare a plan so that you can get the care you want and pay for it in the way that is best for you and your family. Qualifying for Medicaid and some other government benefits can be difficult without spending down all of your assets unless you plan in advance to protect those assets so that they do not need to be spent on your care. There are often benefits available that clients are unaware of. A good elder law attorney can help you determine which programs exist that could help you and whether you may qualify for them now. If you do not qualify for a program now then the attorney should be able to help you plan so that you qualify for the program in the future when you need it.

§ 1.5. A LONG-TERM CARE PLAN

§ 1.5.1. What is a Long-Term Care Plan?

A long-term care plan is a written document that summarizes the issues explored earlier in this chapter. The plan should outline where you want to live as you get older, how you want to be cared for, who will be making medical and financial decisions for you if you cannot make them for yourself, how you anticipate paying for your care, which benefit programs you may qualify for now or in the future, any legal documents that are necessary to execute your plan, and steps that should be taken to protect assets going forward if that is desired.

A good elder law attorney can provide you with this report. If you do a report, please update it every three years because your life will change and the laws will change. It is not enough to do a plan and put it on a shelf. The plan needs to be updated regularly so that it will work as intended when you need it.

For more information, visit the website
of Surprenant & Beneski, P.C. at:
www.the-sb-lawfirm.com.

---

[1] Activities of daily living are generally defined as eating, bathing, dressing, toileting, and ambulating.

[2] Marc A. Cohen, Ph. D., Maurice Weinrobe, Ph.D., Jessica Miller, M.S., & Anne Ingoldsby, MPH, RN, *Becoming Disabled After Age 65: The Expected Lifetime Costs of Independent Living*, (June 2005), AARP Public Policy Institute #2005-08, available at http://assets.aarp.org/rgcenter/il/2005_08_costs. pdf (last visited Nov. 1, 2010).

[3] This document is also known as a "health care proxy and living will" in various states.

CHAPTER 2

SENIOR HOUSING OPTIONS

Henry M. Levandowski, Esquire

Accredited Attorney by the Veterans Administration

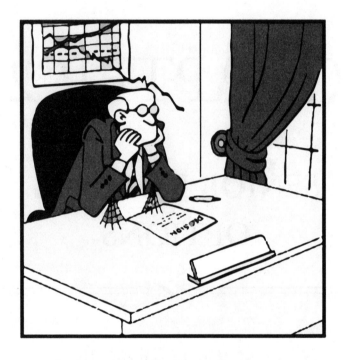

THE PRICE OF DOING NOTHING
IS VERY EXPENSIVE

§ 2.1.
INTRODUCTION:
CONFUSION IN THE
MARKETPLACE

The term "senior housing" can refer to anything from independent living in a retirement community to residency in a nursing home. In between, the marketplace has developed many options as seniors travel along the elder care journey.

Not too long ago, "nursing home" and "retirement home" could have referred to the same facility. Today, there are various levels of "residential care" and "assisted living facilities" available. In fact, over the last twenty years or so, the number and variety of communities and facilities that offer assistance to seniors as they age has multiplied and diversified rapidly. Seniors can now find many combinations of residential accommodations and care services in an ever-increasing variety of settings, with many different pricing plans. Many seniors are not aware of the housing options available to them.

§ 2.2.
TYPES OF SENIOR HOUSING AND RESIDENTIAL CARE

§ 2.2.1. Aging in Place

We all want to live independently for as long as possible. This is the essence of "aging in place." Most often, the phrase is used to mean staying in one's home, even as health circumstances change. Sometimes it can refer to moving to a continuing care retirement community (CCRC), which provides residential services for independent living, assisted living, Alzheimer's or dementia care, and nursing home care. (CCRCs are discussed in § 2.2.4 below. This section covers aging in place in your own home.)

Some of the benefits of living at home as you age are:
- The ability to control your environment;
- Avoiding the trauma of moving;
- Maintaining a comfortable setting for family and friends to gather and offer assistance, if necessary;
- A sense of stability and independence can help preserve mental functioning.

In order to age in place successfully, you must have a plan. Ask yourself:
- What are your health risks?
- What are your financial circumstances?
- Who can you rely on for assistance or caregiving as you age?
- Will you have to hire paid caregivers should you need assistance?

- Are you eligible for any government benefits that help pay for in-home care?
- Do you have, or should you invest in, a long-term care insurance policy that covers in-home care?

Aging in place will probably require modification to the home to accommodate the changes that accompany aging. You may have to install a ramp, handrails, or stair lift, or make a bathroom maneuverable for a wheelchair. These types of modifications will extend the time that you can safely stay at home. You must also anticipate the need for caregivers, either family members or a home health care agency. In most aging-in-place situations, a family member takes care of his or her loved one, at least part of the time. Your planning must address how you will pay for home modifications and caregiving services. Do you have enough income and savings to cover these expenses? Do you qualify for any government benefit programs that help pay for in-home care? Should you consider a reverse mortgage?

Aging in place can be an attractive option to address the vicissitudes of getting older. You will be successful if all the resources at your disposal meet your particular circumstances and desires. Successful aging in place requires a great deal of advance legal and financial planning. Planning earlier rather than later is essential.

§ 2.2.2. Independent Living Communities

Independent living communities are meant for seniors who are healthy enough to maintain their own homes, but desire the services and social interaction afforded by communal living. This type of senior housing can also be referred to as "retirement communities," "senior apartments," "senior housing," or "congregate living." The housing usually consists of an easy to maintain house or private apartment within a community of seniors. Depending on the structure of the particular community, residents may lease or buy their living unit. Independent living communities do not offer health care.

Seniors who choose independent living communities must have the ability to maintain their own residence without need for regular custodial or medical assistance. If such care is needed after moving into a community, residents can hire aides or services of their choice from outside of the community.

The services that may be offered in an independent living community are as follows (note: these services can vary from community to community):

- Recreational, educational, and social activities;
- Communal meals;
- Reading rooms and libraries;
- Transportation services;
- Fitness facilities and activities;
- Swimming pools, golf courses, tennis courts, etc.;
- Beauty salons, barbershops, banks, etc., on site;
- Laundry facilities and services;
- Housekeeping services; and
- Grounds keeping services.

Subsidized housing provided by the U.S. Department of Housing and Urban Development (HUD) offers eligible seniors a low-income housing option. Rent is usually charged as a percentage of the resident's income. The supply of this type of housing can be somewhat limited and long waiting lists are not uncommon. Not surprisingly, there are few amenities provided with low-income senior housing.

An independent living community may be right for you if:

- You are healthy enough to care for yourself and to maintain your house or apartment.
- You are in need of a moderate amount of assistance which can be provided by family or a home health aide.
- You want the safety and security provided by communal living.
- You want the socialization and companionship offered by living among your peers.
- You want the freedom to live independently.
- You want to stop or limit your driving and take advantage of the convenience of the amenities offered by an independent living community.

Given the variety of options available, the costs of independent living communities span a broad range. Subsidized housing is at the low end, while communities where the cost of admission is the purchase of a new home are at the high end. In the middle are communities that rent living spaces and do not otherwise require an entrance fee. There is typically a monthly fee to cover the cost of amenities, management, common utilities, security, etc. A realistic assessment of your financial resources is vital in deciding if an independent living community is right for you.

§ 2.2.3. Assisted Living

Assisted living is the most rapidly expanding type of senior housing. An assisted living facility is a form of senior housing that provides its residents with some assistance with everyday tasks, such as bathing and hygiene, dressing, mobility, and going to the bathroom. Some offer medication assistance as well, depending on state regulation. Meals are usually included along with housekeeping and laundry services. Residents are offered as much independence as possible based on individual circumstances. Housing is typically provided in a studio or one-bedroom apartment in a home-like environment. Some units may have kitchenettes, if it is safe for a resident to use one. Other names for assisted living facility are "personal care home," "boarding care home," "adult congregate care," and "residential care facility."

An assisted living facility will interview and evaluate a prospective resident and his or her family to determine the level of assistance needed, so that an individualized plan of care can be put in place. Subsequently, residents will be evaluated on a regular basis so that services can be customized to needs, which change over time. Typical services offered by an assisted living facility are as follows:

- Monitoring of medical needs;
- Minor medical care;
- Assistance with activities of daily living, as required;
- Housekeeping and laundry services;
- Daily medication management;
- Social and recreational activities;
- 24-hour security;
- Transportation;
- Three meals per day served in a common dining room;
- Around the clock availability of trained staff while maintaining a high level of privacy; and
- Health and exercise programs.

Assisted living costs vary widely depending on the type of housing and the services provided. Customization of care, as reflected in a resident's individualized care plan, means that costs can vary from resident to resident in the same facility. Some assisted living rates are all inclusive, but many assisted living facilities charge a basic monthly rate with add-ons to cover the amount of care and services needed. Assisted living facilities usually do not charge entrance fees.

Assisted living facilities are regulated by the individual state rather than by the federal government. Each state has its own rules and regulations, licensing requirements, and inspection procedures. Therefore, the kinds of care and services that a facility must provide to meet state standards in order to be able to use the title "assisted living" vary across the country.

Assisted living costs are usually paid from a resident's private funds, but there are some notable exceptions. Some long-term care insurance policies cover assisted living. Some states have Medicaid waiver programs that provide Medicaid funding to help with some assisted living costs, for those who are eligible. A veteran who served during wartime may be eligible for VA Aid and Attendance benefits to help pay assisted living costs. Medicare does not cover the services provided in an assisted living facility.

Under certain conditions, part or all of the cost of an assisted living facility can be deducted for federal income tax purposes. Generally, if a resident's physician has prescribed a certain level of custodial and/or medical care, the deduction will apply.

Comparing assisted living facilities based on price can be difficult. Services, amenities, and housing arrangements can vary widely from community to community. It is advisable to have the admissions contract reviewed by an experienced elder law attorney to make sure it is clear what services are being provided for the monthly rate. Also, clarify what the facility's obligation is, if any, if a resident runs out of money.

§ 2.2.4. Continuing Care Retirement Communities

A continuing care retirement community (CCRC) is a type of senior housing that provides multiple levels of residential, custodial, and health care services at one location. At a CCRC, you will find independent living units, an assisted living facility, sometimes a dementia or memory care unit, and a nursing home. A senior usually enters a CCRC as an independent living resident and, in exchange for an entrance fee, is guaranteed on-site assistance with activities of daily living and health care, without having to move elsewhere for the rest of his or her life. Simply put, as a resident's custodial and health care needs change, he or she is able to stay in the same community. The concept especially appeals to couples who, because of the continuum of life-time services, can stay close to each other even if their health needs drastically differ over time.

For independent living residents, amenities are provided that are comparable to those offered in an independent living community, as described above. Just as with independent living communities, the amenities offered by CCRCs vary greatly from community to community.

In addition to the entrance fee, which guarantees the continuum of care for the resident's lifetime, CCRCs charge a monthly fee, as does an independent living community or an assisted living facility. This monthly fee covers amenities and services provided to the resident and can increase as the level of care increases. By opting for a CCRC and entering into a contract upon entry, seniors should not have to worry about where they will live for the rest of their lives, how they will be cared for as they age, and how much it will all cost. In exchange for the entrance fee, the CCRC will provide lifetime services even if the residents should outlive their financial resources.

There are three types of CCRC contracts: (a) extensive, (b) modified, and (c) fee-for-service. With all three, a resident pays an entrance fee and a monthly fee. The "extensive" contract typically provides that a resident is entitled to lifetime care with no increase in the monthly service charge. The cost of this level of protection results in a higher entrance fee, usually a few hundred thousand dollars. This contract usually provides that the entrance fee is non-refundable after a certain number of years of residency. The "modified" contract typically carries a lower entrance fee than the extensive contract. Access to the same level of care is provided but the monthly service charge increases on an as-needed basis. The monthly service charge will reflect a discounted rate compared with the fee-for-service contract discussed below. Also, either a portion or the entirety of the entrance fee may be refundable. The "fee-for-service" contract typically carries the lowest entrance fee, sometimes none at all, and starts with a lower monthly service charge. A resident will be responsible for all care that is needed on an a la carte basis, without the discounts provided for in the modified contract. This means that a fee-for-service resident will pay for assisted living and nursing home care at or near market rates. Seniors opting for the modified or fee-for-service contract should consider obtaining long-term care insurance to help cover the higher monthly service charges. The contracts should be clear about the services covered by the monthly service charge and any other services that are available at an additional cost. The contract should also cover the CCRC's policy regarding the circumstances under which all or a portion of the entrance fee is refundable. Alternatively, it should make clear if the entrance fee is not refundable.

The federal government does not regulate CCRCs. The Continuing Care Accreditation Commission (CCAC), a private non-profit organization, provides voluntary accreditation of CCRCs. CCAC reviews a CCRC's finances, operations, and resident well-being.

Opting to enter into a contract with a CCRC is a major financial commitment on the part of a prospective resident. A senior may spend all or a significant portion of his or her life savings on the entrance fee, which is often in the six figure range. Due diligence requires that a prospective resident explore the financial stability of the CCRC which is relied upon to provide a lifetime of housing and services. Some states require that a CCRC disclose certain financial information to a prospective resident prior to signing a contract. This information can include certified financial statements, balance sheets, escrow and reserve accounts, and how reserve accounts are invested. If your state does not require this level of disclosure, ask for it; any reluctance to provide it should be considered a red flag. It is advisable that the prospective resident and his or her legal and financial advisors thoroughly review this information before any contract is signed. Due diligence can help you to avoid moving into a financially troubled community and avert the risks of unexpected increases in monthly fees and the potential loss of a refundable entrance fee.

Furthermore, an experienced elder law attorney should review the terms, conditions, and requirements of the contract, especially the following:

- Under what circumstances a resident can cancel a contract;
- The refundability of the entrance fee;
- An explanation of all fees and under what circumstances they can be increased;

- A list of all services covered by the monthly service charge and all those available for an extra fee;
- If you outlive your money, does the CCRC have a "benevolence fund" or "resident assistance fund" and are you eligible to access it? If you utilize the benevolence fund, will the CCRC have access to your estate and to what extent?

§ 2.2.5. Nursing Homes

A nursing home is a facility for chronically ill residents who need care 24 hours a day and need more assistance than can be provided at home or in an assisted living facility. Most nursing home care is custodial in nature, but skilled nursing and medical care are also provided. Because of the intensive nature of the care provided, a nursing home is the most expensive type of senior housing.

Admission to a nursing home is based on medical need, as indicated by a doctor's evaluation. Typically, nursing home residents require a combination of assistance with activities of daily living and medical care, usually caused by a severe clinical or cognitive condition. Virtually all nursing home residents will remain there for the remainder of their lives.

Nursing homes resemble hospitals. Residents usually live in a semi-private, hospital-like room and sleep on hospital beds. Nursing home staff are located at nursing stations. A moderate level of medical services is provided, such as staff doctors who make rounds on-site and write orders for needed medications; however, if acute medical care is needed, a resident will be sent to a hospital. Rehabilitative therapy (physical, speech, occupational, etc.) is available. Some nursing homes have lock-down dementia units.

Nursing homes are regulated at both the federal and state levels. In 1987, Congress passed the Nursing Home Reform Act which mandates that nursing homes "must provide services and activities to attain or maintain the highest practicable physical, mental, and psycho-social well-being of each resident in accordance with a written plan of care."

This law and its regulations require that nursing homes:

- Have sufficient nursing staff;
- Upon admission, conduct a comprehensive assessment of each resident's functional capacity;
- Develop an individualized, comprehensive written plan of care for each resident;
- Promote each resident's quality of life and maintain the dignity of each resident; and
- Maintain accurate, complete, and easily accessible clinical records on each resident.

All nursing homes must be state licensed. As part of licensing procedures, state agencies conduct periodic inspections of a nursing home's facilities, staffing, and resident care. The Nursing Home Reform Act requires that the states monitor and enforce the federal standards. Also, states must establish an Ombudsman program to advocate for nursing home and assisted living facility residents to improve their quality of life.

The Nursing Home Reform Act contains other provisions of note:

- A nursing home resident has the right:
  - To choose his or her personal attending physician;

- To receive advance information regarding care
  and treatment options;
- To receive advance information about changes in
  care and treatments which could affect well-being;
- To freely participate in planning care and treatment
  or changes in care and treatment; and
- To accept or refuse any medical treatment or surgery.

- A nursing home's policies and practices regarding
  transfers, discharge, and/or any services provided must
  be identical for all residents regardless of the source
  of payment.

- A nursing home resident is entitled to be reasonably
  accommodated in the receipt of services consistent
  with individual needs and preferences.

- Nursing home admission policies cannot require
  applicants to either waive their rights to, or not to apply
  for, benefits under the Medicaid program.

- Nursing homes cannot require any third party to
  guarantee payment as a condition of admission to,
  expedited admission to, or continued stay in the facility.

- Nursing home residents are entitled to be free from
  any physical or chemical restraint imposed for
  purposes of discipline or convenience and not
  necessary to treat a medical symptom (therefore, vests,
  hand mitts, seatbelts, sedatives, or anti-psychotic drugs
  are prohibited unless ordered by a physician, in writing,
  for an expressly limited period of time).

Nursing home costs can be paid in a number of ways: (a) private
pay; (b) long-term care insurance; (c) Medicare; and (d) Medicaid.

Private pay is paying from your own income and savings for as long as possible. Without consulting an elder law attorney to plan in advance to protect financial resources, most private pay nursing home residents deplete all of their savings and then qualify for Medicaid.

Long-term care insurance may cover all or a portion of nursing home costs. Policies vary greatly from company to company. It is advisable to compare several policies before making a decision to purchase.

It is a common misconception that Medicare pays for long-term care in a nursing home. The truth is that Medicare pays only a small nursing home benefit under very limited conditions. The conditions are that an individual is admitted to a skilled nursing facility for medically necessary rehabilitation care after spending three days in a hospital. A doctor must prescribe the rehabilitation. If these conditions are met, Medicare will cover 100% of the cost for the first 20 days in the skilled nursing facility and somewhat less of the cost for the next 80 days. However, Medicare does not guarantee 100 days of nursing home coverage. Medicare will stop paying for a nursing home resident when the rehabilitation services are determined to no longer be needed, either because the goals of the therapy have been met, or because the resident is not improving under the therapy.

Medicaid is a program jointly funded by the federal government and the states that pays for nursing home care for seniors with limited income and assets. The program is administered at the state level, and there can be significant differences in eligibility rules from state to state. Medicaid has become the de facto long-term care insurance of the middle class; most nursing home residents who do not plan ahead run out of money and then qualify for Medicaid. However, such a result can be avoided by planning in advance with an experienced elder law attorney. For more details on Medicaid and the rules governing Medicaid asset protection planning, see the chapter on Medicaid.

A nursing home has become the senior living option of last resort. It is noteworthy that, while the number of elderly Americans has increased over the last decade, the number of nursing home residents has not. Furthermore, the average age of nursing home residents (and therefore their care needs) are increasing. It would appear that the residential and care alternatives described above are allowing the elderly to put off a nursing home admission until their health deteriorates to a point where there is no other alternative.

§ 2.3.
CONCLUSION

Seniors should plan ahead for their long-term health care needs. The goal should be to select a living option that will provide quality of life and quality of care in a safe environment and be affordable considering available income and resources. Eligibility for government benefits to help pay for long-term care should be explored even in cases where income and assets would appear to be too high. Discuss your options with an experienced elder law attorney.

For more information, visit the website
of Levandowski & Darpino, L.L.C. at:
www.paelderlawnow.com.

CHAPTER 3

REVERSE MORTGAGES

Paul J. Stano, Esquire

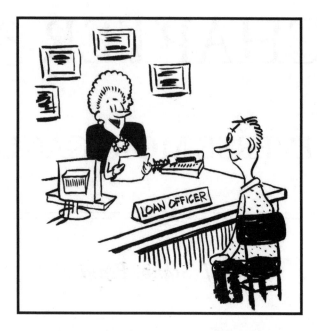

"YOU HAVE AN INTERESTING
CREDIT HISTORY.
I CAN'T WAIT FOR THE MOVIE."

§ 3.1.
WHAT IS A REVERSE MORTGAGE?

A reverse mortgage is a non-recourse loan. In a reverse (or conversion) mortgage, the home is used as collateral to get tax-free cash from the equity of the home without incurring monthly expenses. With a reverse mortgage, the homeowner does not need an income to qualify. There are no income, credit, or health requirements, and there is no effect on Social Security or Medicare benefits.

§ 3.2.
HOW DO REVERSE
MORTGAGES WORK?

To qualify for a reverse mortgage, the homeowner must own the home and be at least 62 years of age, and the home being mortgaged must be the homeowner's principal residence.

The amount of a reverse mortgage is determined by the age of the youngest borrower, the value of the home, and the current interest rate. (Note that older applicants may qualify for larger loans.) With a reverse mortgage, homeowners can pull needed cash from the equity of the home without incurring monthly expenses. The homeowner can receive payments in a lump sum, on a monthly basis for as long as he or she lives in the home, as a line of credit, or any combination of these options.

Once the property is eventually sold – and this can be during the homeowner's lifetime or after his or her death – the sale price of the property pays back the loan and the interest. This rule is in place *even if the sale price is less than the combination of the loan and interest.*

Since the loan is insured by the Federal Housing Administration (FHA), the borrower can never owe more than the value of the home. Lenders must accept *only* the sale price and cannot by law go after the homeowner's other assets.

§ 3.3.
WHAT ARE THE ADVANTAGES OF A REVERSE MORTGAGE?

Lenders cannot force homeowners to sell the property to pay back the loan. Reverse mortgages guarantee that the homeowner can stay in the property for as long as he or she lives in the property as his or her principal residence, pays the property taxes and insurance, and maintains the property in a reasonable condition, *even if the outstanding loan and interest grow to exceed the property's value.*

Only you can decide what a reverse mortgage is worth to you. A reverse mortgage can be a sound strategy to:

- Increase your income
- Pay unexpected expenses
- Pay off debts
- Make necessary changes to your home
- Make your home more accessible
- Help you get the home care services you need to remain independent

Reverse mortgages can be used for:
- Medical bills and prescription drugs
- Long-term health care
- Retirement and estate tax planning
- Daily living expenses

Another important consideration is that any remaining value on the home goes to the homeowner, or his or her heirs, when the house is sold.

§ 3.4.
WHAT ARE THE DISADVANTAGES OF A REVERSE MORTGAGE?

The costs associated with a reverse mortgage are very similar to those of a conventional loan:

- Origination fees
- Inspection fees
- Appraisal and title fees

- Mortgage insurance
- Normal closing costs
- Monthly servicing fees

Reverse mortgage fees can be high, although fees are usually rolled into the loan and not paid up front. A reverse mortgage can cost thousands more than a conventional mortgage. One lower cost option is the FHA reverse mortgage program from the U.S. Department of Housing & Urban Development (HUD).

All reverse mortgages are available in either a fixed rate or an adjustable rate. The fixed rate mortgage must be taken as a lump sum, whereas the adjustable rate may be taken as a credit line or as a combination of a partial lump sum and the remainder as a credit line or regular monthly disbursement. If you choose to receive your reverse mortgage funds as monthly cash payments, these rate adjustments will not change the amount you receive each month. They only affect the amount of interest that is charged on the total loan balance. It's important to calculate the cost of a reverse mortgage against what you would gain, because once you enter a reverse mortgage agreement, the mortgage company may end up with all the equity in the property.

Having a reverse mortgage may offer the ability to take advantage of planning options that require monthly payments which otherwise might not be available to an older homeowner. Be sure that the older homeowner is thinking clearly when considering a reverse mortgage. The prospect of a sudden influx of cash can make it seem as though all of his or her problems will be solved.

Because there are many things to consider, including the possibility of lenders who do not have the homeowner's best interests in mind, it is imperative to get sound advice. The homeowner should discuss his or her reverse mortgage plans with his or her legal and financial advisors and family members before making a decision.

Home ownership is often a person's most valuable asset. It is important to remember that getting a reverse mortgage is essentially the same as you withdrawing the money you would expect to leave to your heirs. For the protection of the homeowner, HUD requires a counseling session with a HUD appproved housing counselor. This can be done by telephone or in person and usually takes about forty-five minutes.

§ 3.5.
WHAT ARE THE RULES
OF REVERSE MORTGAGES?

To reduce their risk, lenders generally limit reverse mortgage loans to amounts that are below their estimate of the property's full value.

Age is an advantage when applying for a reverse mortgage. Borrowers must be at least 62 years old. The older the homeowner is, the more money he or she would qualify for. For example, a 78-year-old borrower would qualify for a larger loan than a 62 year old.

The home must be the principal residence or will be upon its purchase. Qualifying homes include single residences, condominiums, townhouses, apartment complexes up through four units, manufactured homes, Planned Unit Developments, and properties in Revocable Living Trusts.

§ 3.6.
USING REVERSE MORTGAGES TO FUND LONG-TERM CARE

No person should have to sacrifice his or her home or an opportunity for independence to secure necessary health care and supportive services. Most elders who need long-term care would prefer to stay in their own homes. With today's innovative technology and in-home services, this is increasingly possible.

Even severely impaired elders can now continue to live at home if they receive appropriate assistance. Without adequate financial support, however, even modest costs for home care can be prohibitive to many older Americans. The cost of help at home for physically or mentally impaired elders can range dramatically, from an average of $200 per month in out-of-pocket expenses by family caregivers to more than $6,000 per month for elders who need round-the-clock care from home care professionals.

One way to assess the value of a reverse mortgage for long-term care is to determine the planning options available with the proceeds from the mortgage. Because reverse mortgages have relatively high closing costs, this financial tool offers a better value for people who expect to live at home for more than five years. It can be an expensive choice for borrowers who opt for a lump sum and then move out, sell their home, or happen to die within a few years of taking out the loan.

Currently, the reverse mortgage loan becomes due if the last remaining borrower requires care in a nursing home or assisted living facility for more than a year. For severely impaired elders who take out a reverse mortgage, there is a risk that they will not be able to remain at home for many years.

A lump-sum payment will be most helpful for borrowers who are using a reverse mortgage to fund their long-term care. They can use these funds immediately to make major home modifications, pay for a high level of home care services, or utilize estate planning options requiring cash. Borrowers who live alone and lack informal caregivers may also benefit from having a large sum available to pay for professional help at home or to fund their retirement plans (if they have a spouse in a nursing home).

By liquidating their housing wealth through a reverse mortgage, elder homeowners, especially those who are house rich and cash poor, can access a significant amount of cash to pay for long-term care. For example, householders who are dealing with long-term care requirements as a result of Alzheimer's disease can convert a home they own free and clear worth $150,000 into a loan ranging in value from about $60,000 to $100,000, depending on the age of the youngest homeowner. These amounts will fund a significant amount of paid home care to help impaired seniors avoid or delay the need for institutionalization. Borrowers who are less impaired, or who can get some help from family or friends, can significantly increase the amount of time that they might be able to continue to live at home.

Many long-term care users find that their need for care arises slowly, as they gradually require more help with everyday activities at home. For these elders, it may be more appropriate to receive payments from a reverse mortgage through a credit line or tenure payment (which pays for as long as the borrower lives in the home).

§ 3.7.
ESTIMATED DURATION OF FUNDS

A 75-year-old borrower could withdraw from a reverse mortgage line of credit each month. Since long-term care patients who live at home may need assistance for a long time, these amounts can be deducted from a credit line that would last for approximately three to ten years. The amounts that would be available monthly to "impaired" households vary depending on the value of the home.

These funds can have a significant impact on the finances of long-term care patients and their families. By having money of their own to pay for their long-term care, elders can maintain their dignity, as well as retain some independence and control over their lives. For spouses and other family caregivers, these supports can help reduce the financial, emotional, and physical strain that often comes with caring for an impaired elder.

§ 3.8.
REVERSE MORTGAGES AND
LONG-TERM CARE INSURANCE

The equity that most long-term care patients have accumulated in their homes will not be sufficient to pay the entire cost of Alzheimer's care if they require increased levels of assistance, or assistance for a long time. These funds may also be inadequate to meet the needs of couples if both spouses become severely impaired. To shield homeowners from potentially catastrophic costs of long-term care, they need additional resources. One important option is long-term care insurance.

Reverse mortgages can significantly increase the affordability of long-term care insurance. By tapping home equity, homeowners can purchase a policy without having to sacrifice their current lifestyle. There are several options to increase the affordability of long-term care insurance using funds from a reverse mortgage.

One strategy uses the proceeds of a reverse mortgage to pay for insurance premiums. Another approach limits the amount of insurance purchased by elders by increasing the amount of long-term care self-funded through a reverse mortgage. Using a reverse mortgage to pay for long-term care insurance premiums can save current cash assets for other uses.

These three criteria should be met before a reverse mortgage is considered as a source of funds for long-term care insurance:

1. Reverse mortgage borrowers must have insurability to purchase a meaningful amount of long-term care coverage.

2. Payments from a reverse mortgage should pay for a substantial proportion of the insurance premiums, and for any future premium increases. This is particularly important for house rich and cash poor elders who have few other resources with which to pay for coverage.

3. Reverse mortgage proceeds must last long enough to pay premiums until a policyholder needs long-term care; otherwise, a policyholder is at risk of a lapse in coverage without getting any benefits from the insurance.

Each of these criteria raises important issues that need to be addressed about the potential market for this approach and the cost versus value of the benefit to borrowers.

It is difficult to determine how much long-term care coverage a person should purchase. Elders who have Alzheimer's disease, for example, commonly need assistance lasting six years or longer. Other situations and diseases may have different term-of-care requirements.

However, using most of the proceeds from a reverse mortgage to pay for long-term care coverage might be risky for many households. After paying for insurance premiums, they would have little left from their monthly reverse mortgage cash withdrawal to pay for expenses not covered by the $150 per day long-term care benefit or for any premium increases. Since private insurance only pays when policyholders are severely impaired, these homeowners could also face financial problems if they needed help to stay at home prior to triggering their insurance benefits.

For elders with modest amounts of housing wealth, using reverse mortgages for long-term care insurance is not likely to be an option. Single homeowners, age 70, with a home worth $50,000, who use the entire monthly withdrawal from their reverse mortgage line of credit for long-term care insurance, would be able to pay about 80% of the cost of premiums. For couples in this group, cash withdrawals from a reverse mortgage would cover the cost of about 50% of their policy premiums.

Duration of the loan is a critical factor in linking reverse mortgages and private insurance. The risk of needing long-term care increases significantly after age 85. For the typical reverse mortgage borrower who takes out a loan in his or her 70s, this could mean holding onto the loan from five to fifteen years, or longer. Because the reverse mortgage program is relatively new, even experts do not yet have a good understanding of how long reverse mortgage borrowers keep their loans. Preliminary evidence, however, suggests that reverse mortgage borrowers are repaying their loans at a faster rate than would be expected from mortality and move-out rates among older homeowners in general. Further research will be needed to determine the reasons why borrowers terminate their loans and the potential impact this could have on funding long-term care insurance.

Congress passed a provision within the American Homeownership and Economic Opportunity Act of 2000 that encourages the use of reverse mortgages for the purchase of long-term care insurance. Under this law, the U.S. Department of Housing & Urban Development (HUD) is authorized to waive the up-front mortgage insurance premium for reverse mortgage borrowers who use all the proceeds of their reverse mortgage to purchase a tax-qualified long-term care insurance policy.

An analysis of the law suggests that there is likely to be low demand for this financing option. This is primarily due to the lack of overlap in the economic and demographic characteristics of typical reverse mortgage borrowers and long-term care insurance buyers. Implementing this reverse mortgage provision could also present many challenges to HUD. For example, it would be difficult to track whether borrowers are using all the proceeds of their loan to pay for private long-term care insurance.

Use of home equity, particularly through a reverse mortgage, can be an important retirement resource to help impaired elders pay for long-term care services in the home and community. Due to the widespread availability of home equity, using reverse mortgages is an inclusive strategy that strengthens the long-term care safety net for all elders. This is especially important for moderate income elders whose financial needs in retirement often go unaddressed.

Funds from reverse mortgages are available in several payment plans and can be used without restrictions. This flexibility can promote greater consumer direction and choice.

§ 3.9.
CONCLUSION

Tapping housing wealth through reverse mortgages has the potential to fill some critical gaps in our nation's long-term care financing system. Most importantly, by liquidating home equity, seniors impaired by Alzheimer's disease can gain access to an important new source of funding to pay for services and supports at home.

To realize the potential of using home equity for long-term care, we will need to address many challenges. Currently, there is still little awareness of this product among seniors and sufferers of situations requiring long-term care, such as Alzheimer's disease. Many older Americans are reluctant to take out a loan on their homes after having spent many years paying off their mortgages.

Government incentives to reduce the up-front cost of these loans may be able to play an important role in promoting such an approach to financing long-term care. The appropriate use of these funds – whether to purchase services or private insurance – also needs to be examined further to ensure that seniors make wise decisions with their limited housing resources. But with education and counseling, growing numbers of older Americans will be able to continue to live at home with dignity through the use of reverse mortgages.

If you are considering a reverse mortgage, it is important to get as much information as you can and to consider all of your options. For many older homeowners, selling your home and moving to a less expensive home is not always the best way to protect your assets for yourself and your family. However, a reverse mortgage can be just the opportunity that you've been looking for to take care of those substantial long-term care expenses.

For more information, visit the website of
Stano Law at:
http://www.stanolaw.com.

CHAPTER 4

CAREGIVERS

Karol A. Bisbee, Esquire

Registered Nurse

Accredited Attorney by the Veterans Administration

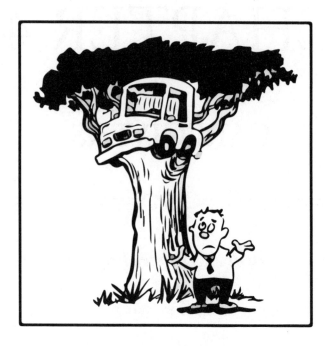

LIFE HAPPENS...
BE PREPARED!

"THE TRUE STRENGTH OF THE AMERICAN FAMILY FINDS ITS ROOTS IN AN UNWAVERING COMMITMENT TO CARE FOR ONE ANOTHER."

– President Barack Obama,
Proclamation, National Family Caregiver's Month, 2009

§ 4.1.
WHAT IS A CAREGIVER?
HOW DID I GET HERE?

**"THERE ARE ONLY FOUR KINDS
OF PEOPLE IN THE WORLD –
THOSE WHO HAVE BEEN CAREGIVERS,
THOSE WHO CURRENTLY ARE CAREGIVERS,
THOSE WHO WILL BE CAREGIVERS
AND THOSE WHO NEED CAREGIVERS."**

– Former first lady Rosalynn Carter

The call comes. It's midnight, or it's 2:00 in the afternoon just as you are getting ready to pick the kids up at school, or just as you are getting ready to leave for an important business trip. The call comes unexpectedly. Mom fell and broke her hip. Dad took a drive and hasn't come home yet. The neighbor tells you there is three days' worth of mail on the porch, Mom answered the door disheveled and confused, and the smell from the house was awful – the neighbor called 911. And, oh, your parents live 850 miles away.

After the shock of the news sinks in, you are thinking, "How quickly can I get there? What will it cost? And what do I have to do to make sure that work, the kids, and the family are all taken care of here?" Then you think, "I didn't know there was a problem;

things weren't this bad; why is this happening now?" And if there are siblings, "Will we deal with this together?"

Welcome to the world of a caregiver. It is the beginning of becoming a family caregiver. You are not alone. As you look around, you may realize that you know many caregivers – a co-worker, a neighbor, another family member, a friend. There are 65.7 million caregivers in the United States, and 14.9 million of them are caring for a loved one who has Alzheimer's disease or another form of dementia.[4]

A family caregiver is an unpaid non-professional who is caring for a family member or friend who is ill or has a disability and cannot live independently. Although most caregivers are female, more men are becoming caregivers. "The average age of caregivers is 48 years."[5] Although, "of those caring for someone aged 50+, the average age of family caregivers is between 50 and 64."[6] A study shows that 64% of caregivers "were employed at some point in the last 12 months," and "on average, caregivers spend 20.4 hours per week providing care."[7] Although for many, when the diagnosis involves Alzheimer's or a related dementia, caregiving is a 24-hour responsibility. A caregiver may be dealing with a variety of illnesses, including stroke, complications of diabetes, cancer, Parkinson's, Multiple Sclerosis, and other chronic conditions that impair an individual's ability to care for himself or herself and live independently. Sometimes, there isn't an illness but simply "old age" and the need for assistance due to the frailties of aging.

Caregiving is a journey. It can be short or long but it carries with it many stresses and the peaks and valleys of joy and depression. Although each caregiving situation is unique, everyone faces similar emotional, physical, and financial concerns.

In my experience, many caregivers are spouses who are 70 years old or older and now need to learn entirely different roles – women who never dealt with the financial issues, and men who never did any of the "women's work" such as dressing and hygiene.

"Regardless of the relationship or diagnosis, family caregivers tend to be selfless in their devotion to the other's well-being. Unfortunately, this selflessness takes its toll on their own health, wealth, and overall welfare," according to Suzanne Mintz, president and CEO of the National Family Caregivers Association (NFCA).[8] Suzanne Mintz further indicates, "most family caregivers won't ask for help." She says that, "For some, it is about privacy and not letting others know the personal details of their lives. For others, it is an admission of failure. But nothing could be further from the truth." Suzanne Mintz also states that, "Family caregiving is more than a one person job and reaching out for help is not a sign of weakness, but rather a sign of strength. It demonstrates a keen awareness of one's own abilities and an understanding that, in order to successfully meet all your responsibilities, whether they are at work, at home, or in the community, you need to rely on others."[9]

§ 4.2.
WHAT'S YOUR STORY:
STAGES OF CAREGIVING

"THE BEST AND MOST BEAUTIFUL THINGS IN THE WORLD CANNOT BE SEEN OR EVEN TOUCHED – THEY MUST BE FELT WITH THE HEART."

– Helen Keller

Perhaps you have read the books, or maybe you've seen an article in a magazine, or read it in a newsletter – the story related by the spouse who is caring for his wife, the story of the mom who is part of the "sandwich generation" caring for her kids and her elderly parent(s), the story of a family member whose life has been completely altered because she is now the primary caregiver for a loved one. It is well known that people find meaning and purpose by telling their stories and having them acknowledged and affirmed. If you search on the Internet, you will find many caregiver stories, and after each is a section for comments where many have responded about how the story has touched their own life situation. You may find that these stories may help you as you travel through the stages of caregiving.

There have been various studies both formal and informal on caregiving and on the stages of caregiving, and the stages are not that different from the stages of grieving. However, I like Dr. Eric Pfeiffer's seven stages for caregivers of individuals who have Alzheimer's or dementia, which certainly also hold true for those caring for individuals who have other chronic illnesses such as stroke or Parkinson's disease.[10]

- Stage 1: Coping with the initial impact of being told the diagnosis.
- Stage 2: To be or not to be – a caregiver?
- Stage 3: At-home caregiving – the long journey.
- Stage 4: Considering institutional placement.
- Stage 5: Caregiving during residential or institutional placement.
- Stage 6: Death of the patient – grief and relief.
- Stage 7: Resuming life – healing and renewal.[11]

STAGE 1: The diagnosis is a life-changing event for many caregivers.[12] At this time caregivers often express their fear of the unknown.[13] There is a tremendous need for information.[14] Information is needed about the disease and its treatments, community resources, government resources, family resources, and the status of siblings and whether there will be cooperation among them. There is a need to know about the loved one's legal and financial status – was preplanning done or is this a crisis? The caregiver and the family become knowledge seekers. They need to ask questions of everyone about everything, including what their role will be as the caregiver, what the risks are for them, and what kind of emotional support is needed from family and friends; they also seek peer support from others who are in the "same boat."[15] This is the stage where you learn how to be a caregiver.

STAGE 2: Initially the role of caregiver is just thrust upon a person.[16] It is important to recognize that not all people are cut out to be caregivers,[17] and that is okay. Even if it is initially thrust upon you, there are alternatives available.[18] Some people are unable to deal with the unfairness of decline and dependence.[19] Some people's personal lives may prevent them from accepting the role; perhaps the relationship with other family members interferes; for some no matter how much they love the person in need, the past relationship may prevent it from working out. An examination of what the role will mean for you and your family is important.

For those who choose this path, the rewards can be tremendous.[20] Aside from knowing that your loved one will get the best care available and a better quality of life as he remains in his own home or in a family member's home,[21] there is also knowing that you will re-establish a relationship that can create memories and shared moments of joy over simple things. For those who decide that they cannot be the primary caregiver, there are options available, such as other family members who may be able to take on the physical care while those who cannot be the primary caregiver provide other support like financial assistance or respite. There are professionals, such as, care managers and aides, who can be hired to take on some of the responsibility.[22]

STAGE 3: Providing care at home is often the longest and most demanding stage.[23] This stage can last from a few months to ten years or many more. There are three sub-stages: mild impairment, middle stage, and advanced stage.[24] In the mild impairment stage, the elder can still be left alone for several hours at a time.[25] In the middle stage, the decline in function or cognition, or both, results in the loss of abilities that demand more of the caregiver's time. It may be difficult to leave the person alone except for very brief periods. In the advanced stage, caregiving has progressed to a 24-hour responsibility, seven days a week.[26] There may be more disruptive behaviors, and the need for respite services is important in order for the caregiver to meet his or her own needs.[27] At this stage, you really need to recognize the signs of caregiver burnout and take the steps necessary to prevent that from happening. Accepting help from others is very important.

STAGE 4: At this stage, the elder may not be aware that he is not in his own home.[28]

STAGE 5: Caregiving does not stop when your loved one enters a nursing home or is otherwise institutionalized.[29] Advocacy and oversight will still be a role. Asking questions and staying informed are still important. You may get more sleep and develop a healthier routine, but there is still a sense of sadness over a loved one's circumstances, and feelings of guilt can be quite strong.[30]

STAGE 6: Knowing that the end will come does not lessen the actual loss, which will still be painful and filled with sadness.[31] Relief from the responsibilities and knowing that someone is "in a better place" do nothing to mitigate the sense of loneliness that can unexpectedly wash over you. Accept that this is part of the normal grieving process. Let others help you.

STAGE 7: In the healing stage you will find ways that can help you move on.[32] Do not deny your experience. Share your experience with others. You may want to find a way to memorialize your loved one. Often people will discover that the experience has left them a changed person – for the better, as they reflect on what their experience has meant to them, to their loved one, and to those around them.

During the initial stages, caregiver's stories are usually about making meaning of the experience. This is often what is most important to them. Caregivers often relate stories about who their loved ones were before and after the appearance of their disease and their eventual decline and what effect it had on the family. The caregiver often wants to establish some continuity between their loved one's past and his current condition as a part of making meaning of the experience. Stories then develop into how the caregiver role is defined and how it changes, involving more emotions about frustration over things that the elder can no longer do and how it can negatively impact the caregiver. For example, when a 70-year-old wife must take on the ill spouse's role, the caregiving wife may find it frustrating and difficult to learn how to do things her husband did, like managing the money or making repairs. Husbands can find it frustrating when they take on the normal "woman's role" in the house. Stories begin to evolve; tips and hints are shared about how to deal with different situations. Feelings of depression can cause the caregiver to feel helpless, which causes the caregiver's own health to suffer. Many stories express frustration regarding day-to-day decisions, about care and the future, which are characterized by uncertainty. Lastly, caregivers tell stories about the need for support and how their lives are on hold because of a lack of resources, support, and finances.

In telling a story or narrative, a person is able to integrate his or her beliefs and make sense of what is happening. This helps to create some order out of the chaos that the illness has created.

What is your story? Read the stories of others, and in your search for information and help, it is likely you will discover that the stories of other caregivers will be similar to your own.

§ 4.3.
THE GREAT DIVIDE:
BARRIERS TO CAREGIVING

"IT REALLY IS THE LONG, LONG GOODBYE."

– Nancy Reagan describing Alzheimer's disease

Family members who care for a person with dementia are at a high risk for serious physical illness, emotional strain, and mental health problems. There are so many things to consider when you embark on the journey as a caregiver. For some, to begin that journey will be an easy decision. For others, it is filled with obstacles.

Siblings can be the biggest source of support, but they can also be the most difficult obstacles. What happens when there are disagreements? When caring for elderly parents, there are unlimited opportunities for disagreements to occur. There can be differences of opinion over money, medical and end-of-life decisions, family possessions, the house or vacation home, and independence and safety decisions, such as living arrangements and whether it is time to take away the car keys. Additionally, is one person shouldering more of the caregiving burden than another? Is one person too controlling or does one person feel left out? Are there too many decision-makers? Are there geographic differences and economic differences? Is there "old baggage" to overcome? There may be distrust of the sibling who has had access to the finances.

"CARING FOR ELDERLY PARENTS
IS SOMETHING THAT SOME OF US
ARE LUCKY TO HAVE AS PART OF OUR LIVES.
I HOPE IT MAKES ME A BETTER PERSON,
A MORE HUMAN PERSON AND ONE
WHO KNOWS THAT SOMEDAY,
THIS MAY BE MY PATH."

– Amy Ball[33]

Even when there aren't any siblings, there are still barriers that caregivers must overcome. They are the same types of barriers that those with siblings face: financial issues, work commitments, fear of getting involved, lack of information, and lack of resources and support.

In addition to this, a caregiver's job can be quite physical. They may have to learn nursing skills, and how to make sure a person doesn't choke. They may need to address behavioral changes or wandering.

Being a caregiver can require putting your own life on hold. For example, saving for your own retirement or child's college tuition may no longer be an option. You may have to quit work or decrease work hours. If your loved one lives a distance from home, there are costs associated with travel.

When considering whether to be a caregiver, some find that the anticipation of grief and loss is too much to overcome. The loved one's loss of independence and self-esteem can have a negative impact on the caregiver's own health. Caregiving is very stressful, and caregivers can experience serious medical issues if they do not care properly for themselves.

§ 4.4.
PROMISE ME YOU'LL NEVER PUT ME IN A HOME: CARING FOR YOURSELF

"SOMETIMES IT HELPS TO KNOW THAT I JUST CAN'T DO IT ALL. ONE STEP AT A TIME IS ALL THAT'S POSSIBLE – EVEN WHEN THOSE STEPS ARE TAKEN ON THE RUN."

– Anne W. Schaef

The words that reverberate in our minds are statements like, "Promise me you'll never put me in a home," or "Why are you making me stay here?" or "Before your dad died, he made you promise to always take care of your mom." These statements have the capacity to cause caregivers feelings of immense guilt. What many caregivers fail to realize in the beginning is that everyone has limits. You can't do it all. Sometimes promises need to be broken to maintain a sense of well-being.

Caregiving is filled with stress and anxiety. It often feels like you are falling into a big black hole filled with uncertainty and fear. Research has shown that children are often the primary care provider for their parents, and feel the additional stress in their lives. There is increased hostility, a decline in happiness, and less autonomy and personal growth. Serving as an advocate can further stress and fatigue.

Be realistic about how much you can do and what you are willing to do. Consider what you are really good at. For example, are you good at researching and getting information, coordinating services and keeping people up to date, making repairs, and/or providing financial assistance? You must know your own limitations and recognize the signs and symptoms of burnout. Listen to the feedback you get from others. Symptoms of burnout may be feelings of depression, a sense of constant fatigue, decreased interest in work, withdrawal from social contacts, use of stimulants/alcohol, increased fear of death, changes in eating patterns, and feelings of helplessness. To cope, join a support group, consult professionals, rotate caregiving with family, exercise, eat healthy, and establish time for yourself.

Anger may be a sign you are overwhelmed. You might feel guilty about almost everything. It is helpful to keep a journal so you can acknowledge your feelings. Make a wish list with the things you need or want, so you are prepared when people ask how they can help.

A caregiver needs patience, tolerance, love, and a sense of humor. It is not unusual to have feelings of exhaustion or for there to be times when you just can't stop crying – when you want your loved one to be like he was before – and when you want or need financial help. Being part of a support group helps to combat feelings of isolation and connects you with others who understand and can offer support. Engaging in personal activities that do not center on the family member who needs care can help increase feelings of caregiver competency and self-worth. Counseling, especially at times of stressful milestones, can be useful.

Contact the local agency on aging and get connected with the many services for the elderly, such as Meals on Wheels, housecleaning, transportation, and social activities. Look to your employer for assistance – some have eldercare programs as part of their benefit program or as an employee assistance program.

These seven caregiver tips and a portion of the explanations following the tips come directly from Christine Jette, RN,[34] and I can't say it better:

1. Get as much help as you can, as early as you can, for as long as you can.

It is normal to feel a full range of emotions as you manage your new role as caregiver. You may love the one who is ill, while still experiencing sadness, anger, or fear. At times you may resent the effect caregiving has on your life. It is common for emotions to fluctuate, and it is important to accept all of these feelings. If you find yourself overwhelmed, reach out to family or friends, or speak with a professional. There are many resources available for caregivers, locally, nationally, and online.

2. Ensuring your own health is the best way to take care of others.

If you are sick or unable to function, you won't be able to look after the people who depend on you for support. Take time to manage your health and to refresh your mind and spirit. Get enough sleep. Eat right. Exercise.

3. Just as you give love to so many, become willing to accept love from others.

Give others the opportunity to take care of you. Ask family and friends to handle tasks such as errands, groceries, rides, housekeeping, laundry, or meal preparation. Family and friends often want to help but they don't know what you need. Tell them! They often feel better because they can help and knowing you can count on others is a relief for you.

4. Your relative may not need (or want) you as much as you think.

From my own experience, I find that the elderly fear the loss of independence and moving out of their own home and into a nursing home, far more than they fear death. With the loss of independence, irritability can set in. The best way to overcome this is to involve loved ones in decisions and give them opportunities to stay involved. Let them continue to use the abilities they have. Remember, they don't have to do things perfectly. As long as their safety is not an issue, let them stay involved, such as making clothing choices for the day, making a sandwich, and performing basic hygiene.

5. Take time for you.

Give yourself permission to maintain your own life as much as possible. Take breaks from caregiving. The empty well has no water to give. Some things you might find helpful: share a takeout meal with others at home or go to a restaurant; pursue a hobby; play cards or board games with family and friends; create a private space in your home to retreat when needed; take time to read a book or magazine before bedtime; listen to relaxing music; soak in the tub. Studies have shown the beneficial effects of pets on a person's overall health. If you have a pet, spend some time with it; if you don't, then go to a shelter to help out; consider bringing a small pet into your home as a foster pet through adoption or purchase.

6. Keep a sense of humor and your perspective.

As they say – laughter is the best medicine. The effect of laughter on good hormones is well known and creates a sense of well-being, while also causing a decrease in stress hormones. Experience something funny each day. Read the comics, watch a favorite light-hearted television show, or read an amusing book. My daughter and I laugh out loud at most *I Love Lucy* shows, no matter how often we have watched them – and at the same time remember my mom and tell stories about her. One genuine laugh a day is all you need to reap its benefits. Laughter is a great tension reliever and healer. While the caregiver role is not funny, you may have situations that on reflection are quite humorous. Remember, none of us are perfect. We make mistakes, learn, and try again. Superwoman lives only in the imagination. You can't do it all, and you will ruin your health trying. Keep a realistic perspective by knowing in your heart that, even on the worst of days, you are doing the very best you can.

7. Join a support group or online community for caregivers.

This will let you know that you are not alone. You will learn coping strategies and meet others who understand what you are going through.[35]

§ 4.5.
LONG DISTANCE CAREGIVING: YOU'RE NOT ALONE

"THESE ARE THE SEASONS OF EMOTION AND LIKE THE WINDS THEY RISE AND FALL . . . UPON US ALL A LITTLE RAIN MUST FALL."

– Led Zepplin

Long distance caregiving brings some unique challenges only because of the distance involved; otherwise, the issues and challenges are the same as they are for any other caregiver. However, there are some hints that can make the caregiving experience easier. When you got "the call," the words you may remember most are "he can't live alone," and those words set in motion the journey of the caregiver.

It's important to remember that you can't do it all at once. Take one step at a time, and remember that you do not need to do it alone. Being far away doesn't mean that you can't be a primary caregiver, it just means it takes more energy and patience. If you can't be the primary caregiver, your role may be that of the person who is able to offer emotional support and respite to the primary caregiver.

Society is much more mobile today than it was a few years ago. Families are scattered all over the world. Living far away requires planning, no matter how long the visit, and even if you don't have a family of your own. You may have a job, a house, plants, a yard, or a pet, and all of these factors need to have forethought before you go away.

Although organization is important for all caregivers, it is even more essential for long distance caregivers. It is essential that you make checklists of your needs. It is helpful to have a list of your strengths and weaknesses so you can identify how others can most effectively help you. When assessing your strengths and weaknesses, ask yourself if you can afford to travel and if you can remain calm and assertive. The ride you are on can be quite bumpy and your emotions may rise and fall like a roller coaster. Will this affect your work, your own kids, your marriage? The demands on the long distance caregiver can be difficult as the caregiver juggles distance and the needs of two households. When you travel, let someone know that you will be away and how to get in touch with you in an emergency.

"MANY OF US CRUCIFY OURSELVES BETWEEN TWO THIEVES, REGRET FOR THE PAST AND FEAR OF THE FUTURE."

– Fulton Orsler

One of the first things you will need to do is gather information about your loved one and about the resources available in the community. Try to build a network in your loved one's community and stay in touch with them on a regular basis. It may be helpful for you to hire a geriatric care manager (GCM) to help coordinate services. These are knowledgeable professionals, usually a nurse or social worker, who specialize in geriatrics.

It is always best when plans are made in advance and legal documents have been put into place. If they haven't, you can still get in touch with an elder law attorney to see what planning and documents can be put into place now, and what benefit options are available.

Each time you visit, assess the safety issues and check that medications and meals are being administered and eaten. Assess whether your loved one is at risk for being taken advantage of financially by scam artists and door-to-door salesmen or telephone marketers.

Check to make sure that you have all of your loved one's important documents: legal name and birth records, social security number and health insurance cards, military records, financial records, property deeds, insurance policies, legal papers, and credit card account numbers.

If you have set up services such as housecleaners or nurse aides, don't be surprised if your loved one accuses them of stealing or moving personal belongings. The elder may become irritated or argumentative. Frequently an elder will not let a provider in the house. The elder might say the provider never showed up or that they were stealing things. This is when a geriatric care manager (GCM) can be particularly helpful. Frequent telephone calls on a regular schedule between you and your loved one will also help.

For each concern that arises, there is an answer and someone who can help you. The key is to know what resources are available and to ASK FOR HELP. You really don't need to do it all alone.

§ 4.6.
TIPS FOR THE CAREGIVER

"THERE ARE THINGS WE DON'T WANT TO HAPPEN BUT HAVE TO ACCEPT, THINGS WE DON'T WANT TO KNOW BUT HAVE TO LEARN, AND PEOPLE WE CAN'T LIVE WITHOUT BUT HAVE TO LET GO."

– Author Unknown

The National Family Caregivers Association has four core messages: believe in yourself, protect your health, reach out for help, and speak up for your rights.[36] Write those messages down and use them to guide you.

As a family caregiver you belong to a very large community. Try to connect with other caregivers for guidance and support. You and your loved one are in this together so just take it one day at a time. Remember that caregiving is always a learning process. Whether the time that you have together is one month or ten years, you will constantly be learning. Often the biggest cause of stress is the feeling that you never have enough information. Identify the resources that can help you find the information and services you need.

Plan before a crisis. Holidays, when families are all together, are a good time to ask some of those important but difficult questions like, "Have you had legal documents prepared by an elder law attorney, especially a durable power of attorney for finances, a health care proxy (durable power of attorney for health care), and a last will and testament?" Have the discussions about all the "what if's." What if you couldn't make health care decisions? Who would you want to make them for you? What if you couldn't handle your money? Who would you want to take care of your finances? What if you were really sick? Where would you want to receive your care? What if Mom or Dad needed someone to care for them, who of the children would be able to participate in the caregiving role? Ask the hard questions in advance so that you have a roadmap for the future. Also, if you have the answers to these questions, and the legal paperwork is in order, then you can act quickly and confidently.

As a caregiver you need to stay flexible because changes can occur daily. You are always "on" but it is important to take regular breaks. You can't just walk away when you are frustrated so you need to take care of yourself to maintain your own health, strength, and patience. Your health is important. If you are not healthy, you can't take care of someone else, so make sure to eat well and get sufficient sleep and exercise. I know that's like a mantra – we hear it everywhere, but when you are in a stressful situation, particularly one that is emotionally and physically stressful, it becomes even more important.

Don't be afraid to ask for help. Participate in a support group with other caregivers. Tap into support services that may be offered through your employer. Use the Internet for information and resources but also for support. There are many online communities for caregivers that share stories and words of advice.

Keep a journal and a three ring binder for information about your loved one. This can be your lifeline of information. You can put anything you want in your binder pertaining to the care of your loved one. It helps you not only to stay focused and organized, but also to

communicate accurately with other care team providers and to artic-
ulate what you need. For example, you can put notes in there about
your loved one's life before and after the illness, family information,
medical information, daily schedule and appointments, medications
and treatments, contact numbers for health providers and other caregivers, emergency numbers for family contacts, lists of agencies, and
any other information you find important to communicate and have
accessible. Take this binder to every appointment. It can be an easy
reference for family, doctors, nurses, therapists, friends, and relatives.
Keep a page protector for business cards and instruction sheets.

Keep a caregiver journal for yourself. A diary of sorts, this can
be a way for you to express your feelings, your hopes, your sadness,
and even your gratitude. You can document motivational sayings and
your feelings when you read them. You can record your sense of loss,
or the wonderful things, such as a great day you had, or your gratitude
for the opportunities the caregiving experience has provided you. The
journal is yours alone as a reminder and an emotional outlet.

Stay in touch with your state and federal representatives and
senators. When you run into a major obstacle, their staff can help
you find information and pave the way to a solution when you can't.
They can't work miracles, but they have access to the rules and people
who know the rules. They can get you the information you need, and
they love to help their constituents.

Caregiving is not just about the physical and emotional care that
you must give your loved one; it is also about building memories.
Spend time visiting with your loved one and sharing stories and
moments that are completely unrelated to the task of caregiving.
Even when your loved one cannot verbally communicate with you,
remember that touch can communicate in many ways that words
cannot. There will be many times when your touch will say everything.

It has been said that a devastating diagnosis can be like a family member who comes for a visit and never leaves. Keep in mind that although caregiving can be difficult at times, it can also be very rewarding. There are good times along with the bad. November is National Caregivers month. During this time, reach out, speak up, and celebrate who you are and what you do with generosity and love, remembering always to take care of yourself.

§ 4.7.
IT'S NOT THE END BUT A BEGINNING: LOSS, GRIEF, AND HEALING

"WHEN YOU ARE SORROWFUL, LOOK AGAIN IN YOUR HEART AND YOU SHALL SEE WHAT IN TRUTH YOU ARE WEEPING FOR, THAT WHICH HAS BEEN YOUR DELIGHT."

– Kahlil Gibran

During the process of caregiving, you may have had a sense of loss – for the life and relationship you had with the other person before you became a caregiver, the loss of financial security, and even the loss of your dreams for the future. Grief can begin before your loved one dies. You may experience some or all of these symptoms:

crying, denial, mood swings, forgetfulness, confused behavior, anger, depression, and loneliness. You may also have health symptoms such as weight gain or loss, sleep problems, nervous behavior, and general fatigue. Fatigue and stress can lead to depression, which is treatable. You may experience an exacerbation of symptoms for other chronic diseases, such as flare ups of your diabetes or chest pain.

"DEATH LEAVES A HEARTACHE NO ONE CAN HEAL, LOVE LEAVES A MEMORY NO ONE CAN STEAL."

– From a headstone in Ireland

Sometimes letting go simply means accepting what is and being the best that you can be. Sometimes letting go means moving your loved one out of his or her (or your) home and into a facility. This is not a failure on your part, but a realization of what is best for your loved one given the circumstances. You will still be a caregiver as you oversee and advocate for your loved one's best care, visit him, and keep him in your heart, helping him to have the best quality of life possible.

Being a caregiver is a big responsibility, and it can be isolating. Frequently it is a long and challenging journey. Most days, one person is the center of your universe. You are the information gatherer, physical caregiver, money manager, coordinator of services, child, spouse, and so much more – all the while trying to continue that special relationship defined through love with the person who is so different from the way he or she was.

During the process of caregiving, many begin to experience a sense of loss and grief. When your loved one passes away, it is not unusual to feel the pain of loss, sometimes even years later. This can be especially true around the holidays and those times that were special to you and your loved one. Grief is normal, and generally healing occurs gradually. There will be good days and bad days. There will be days when you may be angry with everyone. You might feel guilty that you aren't a good caregiver. You may blame yourself for past missteps. You might feel guilty about feeling angry and have a sense of overwhelming sadness with periods of crying and such feelings of loneliness, emptiness, and despair. You may even become clinically depressed. Grief and caregiver stress can lead to physical illness, exhaustion, insomnia, headaches, and more, but with acceptance comes hope for the future, peace, and a sense of purpose. Not everyone feels grief immediately. It can come years later.

Give yourself permission to cry. Tears can be a tremendous emotional release, but be careful about letting yourself stay sad and tearful for long periods of time. Reach out to others for help. There isn't a right or wrong way to grieve. Grief is like the roller coaster we mentioned before. One minute you are fine and then something happens that triggers the guilt and feelings of hopelessness. Grieving never really ends. It just becomes a lesser form of sadness. Never forget nor want to forget about a life that was important to you.

Make the most out of moments with your loved one. Focus on the positives. A wise person told me to remember my parents by talking about them. Through stories and relived memories, both good and bad, will come laughter, and it will keep them alive. They will always be in your heart, and they will always be a part of you, and whether it brings tears to your eyes or a smile to your lips, it does not matter, for you will move on, and they will be there with you.

Healing is a process as well. For it to occur, you must allow yourself to feel both your pain and joy. Talk to family and friends or write in a journal. Let them into your world. Join a support group. Do the usual things, get plenty of sleep, eat healthy, and exercise. It helps to share family stories with your children about their grandparents, or with your siblings and other relatives about your parents or loved one – remember their lives and how they influenced your life. Go through family albums with your children and family members and the stories will start flowing. Know that there will be difficult times, especially at the holidays and special times. Be good to yourself and do the things you enjoy; that is what your loved one would have wanted for you.

For more information, visit the website of the
Law Office of Karol Bisbee, P.C. at:
http://bisbeelaws.com.

[4] Used with permission of Family Caregiver Alliance: National Center on Caregiving, *Fact Sheet: Selected Caregiver Statistics*, at http://www.caregiver.org/caregiver/jsp/content_node.jsp?nodeid=439 (last visited Sept. 17, 2011) (citations omitted). For more information, visit http://www.caregiver.org or call (800) 445-8106.

[5] *Id.* (citation omitted).

[6] *Id.* (citation omitted).

[7] *Id.* (citations omitted).

[8] Used with permission from Allsup & National Family Caregivers Association, *Message to Family Caregivers: "Reach Out for Help"* (Oct. 29, 2010), at http://www.prweb.com/releases/ALLSUP/NFCA/prweb4718994.htm (last visited Sept. 17, 2011).

[9] *Id.*

[10] Eric Pfeiffer, *Stages of Caregiving*, Am. J. Alzheimer's Disease and Other Dementias, vol. 14 no. 2, pp. 125-27, Copyright © Mar./Apr. 1999 by SAGE Publications, available at http://aja.sagepub.com/content/14/2/125 (last visited Sept. 28, 2010). Reprinted by Permission of SAGE Publications.

[11] These seven states of caregiving were taken verbatim from Eric Pfeiffer, *Stages of Caregiving*, Am. J. Alzheimer's Disease and Other Dementias, vol. 14 no. 2, pp. 125-27, Copyright © Mar./Apr. 1999 by SAGE Publications, available at http://aja.sagepub.com/content/14/2/125 (last visited Sept. 28, 2010). Reprinted by Permission of SAGE Publications.

[12] Eric Pfeiffer, *Stages of Caregiving*, Am. J. Alzheimer's Disease and Other Dementias, vol. 14 no. 2, pp. 125-27, Copyright © Mar./Apr. 1999, available at http://aja.sagepub.com/content/14/2/125 (last visited Sept. 28, 2010). Reprinted by Permission of SAGE Publications.

[13] *Id.*
[14] *Id.*
[15] *Id.*
[16] *Id.*
[17] *Id.*
[18] *Id.*
[19] *Id.*
[20] *Id.*
[21] *Id.*
[22] *Id.*
[23] *Id.*
[24] *Id.*
[25] *Id.*
[26] *Id.*
[27] *Id.*
[28] *Id.*
[29] *Id.*
[30] *Id.*
[31] *Id.*
[32] *Id.*

[33] Used with permission from Tender Loving Eldercare, *Do You Have Patience with Your Aging Parents?*, cmt. posted Jan. 16, 2010, at http://tenderlovingeldercare.com/do-you-have-patience-with-your-aging-parents (last visited Feb. 3, 2011).

[34] Used with permission from The Grieving Heart, *Caring for the Caregiver*, at http://www.thegrievingheart.info/caringforthecaregiver.html (last visited Feb. 3, 2011).

[35] The seven caregiver hints and portions of their descriptions come directly from Christine Jette, RN. Used with permission from The Grieving Heart, *Caring for the Caregiver*, at http://www.thegrievingheart.info/caringforthecaregiver.html (last visited Feb. 3, 2011).

[36] Used with permission from National Family Caregivers Association, *About NFCA*, at http://www.nfcacares.org/about_nfca/ (last visited Sept. 17, 2011).

CHAPTER 5

MYTHS AND MISUNDERSTANDINGS

Janis A. Carney, CELA

Certified Elder Law Attorney by the
National Elder Law Foundation

Certified Specialist Estate Planning Trust and Probate Law by
the State Bar of California Board of Legal Specialization

Accredited Attorney by the Veterans Administration

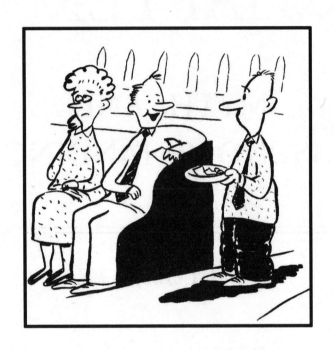

"DO YOU TAKE COUPONS?"

§ 5.1.
ON MATTERS OF
ESTATE PLANNING

§ 5.1.1. Only Rich and Old People Need an Estate Plan

FALSE. Estate planning is important for everyone, rich or poor, young or old. Estate planning includes much more than planning to save taxes for the wealthy or planning for the disposition of your estate when you are very old. People of all ages have accidents or suffer sudden illnesses and could die or become severely incapacitated with little or no warning. Estate planning provides for the disposition of your assets according to your wishes. It includes your instructions regarding who should care for you or for young children if you cannot do so yourself and lack the mental capacity to make decisions. It allows you to say who should handle your finances and whether a court or someone else should review that person's management. It makes sure that you have thought through what will become of all of your assets and that you have a coordinated plan for everything. Estate planning is an ongoing process with the parts needing to be updated as your life's story unfolds over the years.

§ 5.1.2. Estate Planning Is No Big Deal;
I Can Do It Myself

TRUE AND FALSE. Of course you can do some simple estate planning on your own. There is a lot of information you can access from books and on the Internet about estate planning, and there are forms from kits you can use to create your own documents such as living trusts, last will and testaments, advance health care directives, living wills, and powers of attorney. However, most form documents are not state specific and may not meet your state's requirements for validity. They also may not include provisions that are important in your situation, or they may include conflicting and ambiguous provisions. An estate plan is much more than merely creating a set of documents. It requires knowing what those documents should say in a particular case and how they will work when they are needed. Estate planning documents created from a kit are a leading cause of estate and trust litigation. They can destroy relationships when your loved ones fight over their interpretation and often cost thousands of dollars to fix.

§ 5.2.
ON THE SUBJECT OF PROBATE

§ 5.2.1. Having a Will Avoids Probate

FALSE. This is one of the most common misconceptions. The truth is that a Will is a one-way ticket to Probate. Probate is a formal court process by which it is determined whether a Will is valid. In most states, the Probate proceeding also provides notice to the beneficiaries under the Will as well as to the decedent's heirs as defined under the state's rules and to potential creditors who are owed money by the decedent. How complex the Probate proceeding will be depends on your state's rules, the size of your estate, and to whom you leave your estate. Minor children cannot take possession of property or money left to them; so not only must your Will be probated, but the assets left to a minor child will probably require a court supervised Guardianship to protect the child's inheritance as long as the child is a minor.

§ 5.2.2. Having a Living Trust Avoids Probate

TRUE AND FALSE. It is true that in most states, assets held in a Living Trust do not have to go through Probate. Unfortunately, many people who create a Living Trust fail to transfer title to all of their assets to the trust, resulting in assets passing under their Will instead. Even when all of a person's assets are in a Living Trust, there may be circumstances that require a Probate or Probate-like proceeding anyway, such as litigation over some of the assets or a court contest to determine the validity or meaning of the trust.

§ 5.2.3. Probate Is Expensive

TRUE AND FALSE. The cost of a formal Probate is determined under each state's laws and generally includes attorney's fees, executor's fees, court filing fees, and miscellaneous costs. In some states attorney's fees and executor's fees are a set percentage of the value of the estate, and in other states the attorney and executor may charge reasonable hourly fees that are subject to court approval. Further, the executor will often waive his/her fee if he/she is a relative or close friend of the family. Finally, many costs that make a Probate seem "expensive," such as preparing an accounting, litigating claims, and paying taxes, are not the result of the Probate proceeding itself but may arise in any type of estate administration.

§ 5.2.4. Avoiding Probate Saves Taxes

FALSE. Probate and estate or inheritance taxes are not connected. Probate is merely the court proceeding set up by your state to determine the validity of your Will and supervise the administration of your estate. While Probate may incur fees and costs as discussed in the question above, taxes are not part of them. Estate and inheritance taxes are determined by completely separate federal and state laws and are based on the size of your estate and to whom you left it, not on whether or not there is a Probate.

§ 5.3.
MORE ABOUT WILLS

§ 5.3.1. My Spouse Will Automatically Get Everything When I Die if I Don't Have a Will

TRUE AND FALSE. Depending on the state where you live when you die, if you do not have a Will, your estate will be divided between your surviving spouse and your children or parents. If you live in a community property state like California, all community property assets will go to your surviving spouse and any separate property will be split between your spouse and your children or parents.

§ 5.3.2. I Must Have a Will or the Government Will Take Everything When I Die

FALSE. If you die without a Will, the laws in the state where you resided at the time of death provide for the disposition of your estate to your heirs (typically your next of kin). Depending on the state laws where you lived, your estate may go all to your surviving spouse or may be split between your surviving spouse and your children or parents. In some states, registered domestic partners have the same or similar inheritance rights to those of a surviving spouse.

Only in those very rare cases where someone has absolutely no living relatives, even very remote ones, does the property go to the state if the decedent died without leaving a Will or trust, or naming someone as a beneficiary on an account.

§ 5.3.3. A Simple Will Takes Care of Everything

TRUE AND FALSE. A simple Will *can* control who gets your estate, but often does not. Many assets, such as life insurance, annuities, retirement accounts, and even some bank accounts may have beneficiaries designated who will get those assets directly from the insurance company or financial institution. In addition, you may have named someone as a *joint tenant with rights of survivorship* on your property or account who will take that property or account automatically when you die.

§ 5.3.4. When I Die, a Lawyer Will Have to Read My Will to My Family

FALSE. This is a misconception born out of the movies. In fact, it is very rare for an attorney to meet with the decedent's entire family to formally "read the Will" to them. Rather, the executor's attorney will usually meet with and explain the terms of the Will only to the executor as part of the discussion about the Probate process and other administration issues, such as taxes. The decedent's family members and other beneficiaries will receive a copy of the Will as part of the Probate process that they usually read for themselves.

§ 5.4.
ALL ABOUT LIVING TRUSTS

§ 5.4.1. Everyone Needs a Living Trust

FALSE. Although a Living Trust may have many advantages, not everyone needs one. Property can also pass without Probate by utilizing beneficiary designations, joint tenancies, and small estate proceedings. However, a Living Trust may be best for an estate that will be subject to federal estate or state death taxes, that holds extensive investments or real estate, that leaves assets to minor children or to children who have a disability, that involves a second marriage, or in instances where creditor protection is desired.

§ 5.4.2. Only Rich People Need a Living Trust

FALSE. A Living Trust is designed to authorize someone you designate as "trustee" to administer your trust estate after you die in accordance with the trust terms without having to go through Probate. Since Probate avoidance is a major goal and advantage of a Living Trust, estates that would not require a Probate, such as where the estate is below the dollar value that requires Probate in your state, would not need a Living Trust either. However, there are other reasons besides avoiding Probate to have a Living Trust, including creditor protection and continuing administration of the estate of a minor. Depending upon your state's laws, privacy and costs of administration may be additional advantages of a living trust.

§ 5.4.3. If I Have a Living Trust, Nothing Needs to Be Done When I Die

FALSE. Although a Living Trust will generally avoid Probate, it still must be properly administered. Trust property must be valued, taxes must be filed and paid, debts and expenses must be paid, and the assets must finally be distributed according to the terms of the trust. It is important that the trustee get legal advice in order to make sure that all of the legal requirements are taken care of before the trust estate is distributed to the beneficiaries. If something comes up after the assets are distributed, the trustee could be held personally liable for making it right, as once a beneficiary gets an asset it may be impossible to get it back.

§ 5.4.4. A Living Trust Avoids Estate Taxes

TRUE AND FALSE. A Living Trust does not automatically avoid estate taxes. However, in some cases, especially for wealthy married couples, a properly drafted Living Trust for a married couple can do some tax planning by providing for the assets owned by the first deceased spouse to stay in a Marital Trust for the spouse, deferring the estate taxes on those assets until the surviving spouse's death. The Living Trust may also set up a ByPass Trust to avoid being estate taxed on the surviving spouse's death on the amount of the deceased spouse's estate that would be exempt from estate tax. A properly drafted Will can also create these trusts, although a Will is subject to Probate while a Living Trust is not. However, a Marital Trust and a ByPass Trust are now not the only ways to accomplish savings or deferring estate tax at the first spouse's death. A surviving spouse also may now claim his/her deceased spouse's estate tax exemption amount and add it to the surviving spouse's own exemption amount. The requirement of this new rule, called "portability" are technical and include filing a timely estate tax return for the deceased spouse's estate and making an election to claim the deceased spouse's unused exemption amount. Anyone considering using portability should see the advice and assistance of any estate planning, elder law, or tax attorney or other qualified tax professional, such as a CPA.

§ 5.5.
SOME OTHER THOUGHTS ON TAXES

§ 5.5.1. I Can Give Everything Away Before I Die to Avoid Estate Taxes

TRUE AND FALSE. It is possible to give away everything before you die and avoid estate taxes on your death. However, the value of gifts made within three years of death in anticipation of death can be brought back into your estate for estate tax purposes. In addition, there may be other tax consequences on gifts such as federal and state gift taxes, local fees on transfers of real property, and income taxes on gifts of funds from a retirement account.

§ 5.5.2. I Am Income Taxed on Anything I Receive by Gift or Inheritance

FALSE. Gifts and Inheritances are not income to the recipient and, thus, not subject to income taxes when received. Naturally, once the gift or inheritance is received, the recipient is responsible for the income taxes on the earnings produced by the assets gifted or inherited. In addition, if the asset inherited is a deferred income account, such as an IRA, on which income taxes have never been paid, then when the funds are withdrawn from that account, the recipient will owe income taxes on them.

§ 5.5.3. I Can Only Give Away $14,000 a Year Tax-Free

FALSE. The general rule is that each person may currently give away up to a total of $5.43 million dollars (in 2015) gift tax free during his/her lifetime or upon his/her death, or a combination of both. This is called the unified gift and estate tax exemption amount. However, the donor of such lifetime gifts (to the extent they exceed the annual gift tax exclusion amount, discussed next) must file a gift tax return, due by April 15th of the year following the gift. In addition to the unified exemption amount, a person may make gifts each year to each and every person to whom the donor desires to make them, not just to his/her family, of up to that year's annual gift-tax exclusion amount, which is $14,000 for 2015. These annual exclusion gifts do not require a gift tax return to be filed. Both the unified exemption amount and the annual exclusion amount increase annually based on the cost of living adjustment. However, the rate for the annual exclusion goes up only in $1,000 increments. So, it may take several years to accumulate sufficient cost of living adjustments to push the annual exclusion up to the next $1,000 level.

§ 5.5.4. Life Insurance and IRAs Pass Tax Free When I Die

TRUE AND FALSE. The proceeds from all life insurance and retirement accounts you own when you die are included in your taxable estate for federal estate tax purposes. However, life insurance on your life that is owned by someone else, such as your surviving spouse or child, or that is held in a properly designed and administered Irrevocable Life Insurance Trust, is not in your taxable estate and will not be subject to estate taxes. Life insurance is not taxable income while IRA distributions are taxable income when withdrawn from the account. Life insurance may not be subject to state inheritance taxes depending upon your state's laws.

§ 5.6.
ON LONG-TERM CARE PLANNING

§ 5.6.1. Medicare Pays for Long-Term Care

FALSE. Medicare (not Medicaid) is health insurance paid for by deductions taken from your salary during your working years. It covers expenses related to your health in order to make you well. As such, it will cover the cost of a nursing home for a short time if needed for you to get well, such as in order for you to get comprehensive rehabilitation. However, as soon as you are deemed to no longer be improving, Medicare will stop paying for the nursing home. In addition, Medicare will only pay for a nursing home for up to 100 days, subject to a substantial co-payment after day 20.

§ 5.6.2. If I Go on Medicaid, the State Will Take My House and All of My Assets

FALSE. When you enter a nursing home all you owe is the monthly fee for services. If you are unable to pay that fee either privately or through insurance, you may qualify for Medicaid to pay it for you. However, federal law requires the state to try to recover the cost of the Medicaid services you received from your estate upon your death. The amount that the state can recover is limited to "the lesser of" the amount the state paid for your care on Medicaid or the value of your estate at the time of your death. There are circumstances where the state is unable to recover even when there are assets in your estate to pay, such as where you leave a surviving spouse or a disabled or blind child, or where the recovery would result in a substantial hardship on someone who cared for you before you went into the nursing home. The criteria for hardship waivers are left to the states to determine.

§ 5.6.3. Medicaid Allows Me to Give Away $10,000 a Year

FALSE. Medicaid has no safe harbor amount that may be gifted during the look-back period without consequences; although in some states, it is currently still possible to make small gifts without any penalty attaching to them. Again, check with an elder law attorney in your state before making gifts if Medicaid will be needed in the foreseeable future.

§ 5.6.4. I Have to Spend or Give Away Everything to Get on Medicaid

FALSE. The Medicaid program allows you to continue to own certain "exempt" assets and other assets that are "unavailable" to you and still qualify for Medicaid. The primary exempt asset is your home. There are some differences between the states in the exempt assets and what will be treated as unavailable so you should seek the advice of an elder law attorney in your state.

§ 5.6.5. I Have to Wait 5 Years after Giving Anything Away Before I Can Get Medicaid

TRUE AND FALSE. The "5 year look-back rule" refers to the how far back Medicaid can look to find any gifts you made in anticipation of qualifying for Medicaid to pay your long-term care. If you made gifts during this period, then Medicaid will assess a penalty period, based on the value of the gift(s), during which time Medicaid will not pay for your care. If you give away substantial assets as part of your long-term care planning, then it may be necessary for you to wait until the 5 year look-back period has lapsed before applying for Medicaid. However, when this penalty period begins and how it is calculated varies from state to state. Due to the complexity of the rules, it is strongly recommended that you seek advice from an elder law attorney in your state before making gifts as part of a long-term care plan.

§ 5.6.6. A Living Trust Protects My Assets if I Need Medicaid

FALSE. The assets held in your Living Trust will be deemed available and countable in determining your eligibility for Medicaid to pay for long-term care in a skilled nursing facility.

§ 5.6.7. If I Go into a Nursing Home on Private Pay, the Nursing Home Can Evict Me When I Qualify for Medicaid

FALSE. Federal law prohibits a nursing home from evicting patients other than for a very select list of reasons and qualifying for Medicaid is not one of them. So, as long as the nursing home is a qualified Medicaid facility, it cannot discriminate against you on the basis of your source of payment for care. The nursing home may not be happy that you are now on Medicaid and you may feel like they are trying to kick you out. However, actually serving you with an eviction notice on the basis of Medicaid being the source of your payment for care is illegal.

§ 5.6.8. A Pre-Nuptial Agreement Protects My Spouse's Assets if I Need Medicaid

FALSE. A pre-nuptial agreement has no effect on eligibility for Medicaid. Medicaid counts all of both spouses' assets in determining eligibility for Medicaid. However, in some states, a spouse's refusal to pay for care or to sell an otherwise countable asset may cause the spouse's assets to be treated as "unavailable" for Medicaid eligibility purposes.

§ 5.6.9. I Don't Need a Lawyer for Medicaid Planning

FALSE. Medicaid is a federal program administered by the states. As such, the federal rules are interpreted in each state according to its laws, rules, and regulations. In some states, the program is even being administered under "draft regulations," meaning that they have never been officially enacted and, so, are not part of that state's official code of regulations. Also, because Medicaid rules differ somewhat from state to state, there are few books or other publications detailing the rules and those that do exist may not apply in your jurisdiction. You should seek the advice of an elder law attorney in your state regarding your Medicaid planning

For more information, visit the website of
Carney Elder Law at:
www.carneyelderlaw.com.

CHAPTER 6

ALZHEIMER'S AND PARKINSON'S DISEASE: WHAT PATIENTS AND THEIR FAMILIES NEED TO KNOW

Dennis J. Toman, CELA

Certified Elder Law Attorney by the
National Elder Law Foundation

Board Certified Specialist in Elder Law,
Estate Planning and Probate by the
North Carolina State Bar

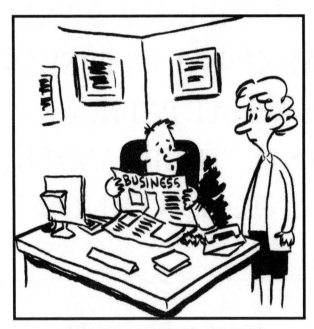

"COMPLETING A MEDICAID APPLICATION
IS LIKE LISTENING TO MY TEENAGER.
I DON'T UNDERSTAND EITHER OF THEM."

§ 6.1.
THE CHALLENGE OF FACING ALZHEIMER'S AND PARKINSON'S DISEASE

Alzheimer's disease and Parkinson's disease are two types of debilitating illnesses that slowly rob a person of his or her physical and mental abilities. Often after years of suffering with the disease, the person reaches the point where he or she no longer can provide his or her own care or make his or her own decisions, or even attend to the most basic human functions. Not only do these prolonged illnesses drain the individual's physical and mental abilities over time, but the individual's loved ones must bear a burden no matter how willingly borne, that weighs them down year by year, then by the month, and finally by the day and minute.

Adding further insult is the astounding cost of paying for care for a person in the later stages of Alzheimer's or Parkinson's. And with the prospect of declining capabilities and increasing costs come important legal decisions and planning strategies to prepare and plan for likely future medical and financial needs.

This chapter is intended to help explain and clarify critical legal issues faced by those who have Alzheimer's or Parkinson's disease and by their loved ones. A word of caution applies, however, because many of the laws and financial issues certainly will change over time and vary by state. For the best advice for your own planning situation, consult an experienced elder law attorney in your state.

§ 6.2.
WHAT DOES IT MEAN TO HAVE ALZHEIMER'S OR PARKINSON'S DISEASE?

Alzheimer's disease is the most common type of dementia, affecting approximately 5.2 million Americans, and it is the sixth leading cause of death in the United States.[37] This disease of the brain progressively impairs behavior and personality, while causing problems with memory, thinking, and judgment. Symptoms usually develop and worsen over time, eventually interfering with daily tasks.[38] According to the Alzheimer's Association, "those who have Alzheimer's live an average of eight years after their symptoms become evident, but survival can range from four to 20 years, depending on age and other health conditions."[39] There is no cure for Alzheimer's but current treatments can temporarily slow the progression of the symptoms.[40] Alzheimer's is not a normal part of the aging process, although most people who have Alzheimer's are over age 65.[41] However, up to 5% of those who have Alzheimer's have "early-onset Alzheimer's," often in their 40's or 50's.[42]

Parkinson's disease is a motor system disorder, resulting from the loss of brain cells that produce the chemical dopamine.[43] Dopamine allows the brain to transmit signals to produce smooth movement of muscles. Loss of dopamine causes neurons to fire without normal control, resulting in the person being less able to direct or control his or her movement.[44] These motor control symptoms of Parkinson's are familiar to most people as tremor (or trembling) in hands, arms, legs, jaw, and face; rigidity or stiffness of the arms, legs, and trunk; bradykinesia or slowness of movement; and impaired balance and coordination called postural instability.[45] Parkinson's also has "non-motor" symptoms, including cognitive impairment ranging from mild memory loss to dementia, and depression and anxiety.[46] Parkinson's symptoms affect patients differently. Not all patients experience all of the symptoms, and the rate at which the symptoms worsen varies, too.[47]

The average age of onset for Parkinson's disease is 60, but the disease can strike as early as age 18.[48] An estimated 1 million people in the United States, and between 4 and 6 million worldwide, have Parkinson's.[49] There is no cure for Parkinson's currently, and the types of treatment depend upon the symptoms evidenced by the particular patient.[50]

§ 6.3.
CRITICAL CONCERNS:
LEGAL, FINANCIAL, AND CARE

Having a loved one with Alzheimer's or Parkinson's disease poses many challenges. What types of treatment and care are best? How do you deal with constant worry over what will happen next? How can you take care of your loved one who has Alzheimer's or Parkinson's while taking care of yourself? Can your loved one remain at home, and if not, where will he or she get care? And, the ever present question: if your loved one eventually needs care at a nursing home, how can you pay for it without going broke?

As you proceed through this chapter, you will learn more about the planning steps, strategies, documents, and key concerns your elder law attorney may consider for you or your loved one who has Alzheimer's or Parkinson's. As you travel this path, keep in mind that

Alzheimer's and Parkinson's affect people in different ways; everyone's situation is unique, and no "one size fits all" approach applies.

§ 6.3.1. Diagnosis and Treatment

Many uncertainties surround the diagnosis of Parkinson's and Alzheimer's. Both diseases are chronic (meaning they persist over a long period of time) and progressive (meaning their symptoms grow worse over time). However, not everyone experiences the same symptoms or progresses at the same rate. For example, not all Parkinson's patients eventually experience dementia, although it sometimes happens in later stages.

For people worried about memory loss, declining physical abilities, and/or behavior changes, consulting with a doctor for an early diagnosis has many advantages, including the following:

- More time to make choices that provide quality of life;
- Less anxiety about suspected but unconfirmed disability;
- Narrowing the diagnosis and having a better chance to benefit from treatment; and
- More time and ability to plan for the future.

After diagnosis, treatment depends on your doctor's recommendations. But just as importantly, you should seek out information, understanding, and guidance from others who have travelled this path before you, and who daily live with or assist those with these diseases. Becoming involved with support groups and resources offered through the local chapters for Alzheimer's and Parkinson's disease can be an important lifeline as the disease progresses over time.

§ 6.3.2. Prompt Planning for
Legal and Financial Concerns

By acting in the early phases of Alzheimer's and Parkinson's disease, patients can ensure that their wishes concerning financial and health care matters are known and followed when they can no longer speak or make their own decisions. Because the progression of both diseases is unpredictable, proper legal documents should be put in place as soon as possible. Having proper legal planning and documents allows more flexibility, better equipping patients and their families to deal with whatever legal, medical, or financial problems happen later.

§ 6.4.
NAMING SOMEONE TO MAKE DECISIONS FOR YOU IF YOU NO LONGER CAN DO SO

Many Alzheimer's and Parkinson's patients face a future when they can no longer make their own decisions. Proper planning allows you to name a family member or trusted friend to have the legal authority to carry out your wishes if you can no longer make or communicate your own wishes. But if you don't grant these decision making powers yourself, someday your family may be forced to pursue a court appointed guardianship or conservatorship. As discussed below, generally a guardianship limits planning options, and it is more expensive, time-consuming, and difficult than using a power of attorney.

Planning tip: If you or a loved one is faced with a diagnosis of Alzheimer's or Parkinson's, the single most important planning step is to put into place the correct powers of attorney for financial and medical decisions. All too often I see clients who have no powers of attorney at all, or who had "traditional" powers of attorney that were not written with elder care concerns in mind. I shudder every time I see a "form" power of attorney purchased online or at an office supply store, because in my experience they are often deficient in dealing with these situations and are no substitute to having a carefully crafted power of attorney from a consultation with an elder law attorney. Having a "weak" power of attorney severely limits planning options. It may place your entire estate at risk for long term care and nursing home costs, possibly leaving you out of money and out of options at one of the most frail and vulnerable times of your life. Don't let this happen to you or your loved ones! Talk with an experienced elder law attorney to make sure you have the proper powers of attorney in place to protect yourself and your family.

§ 6.4.1. Managing Financial Matters: The Durable Power of Attorney

A durable power of attorney is a document that names an agent to handle financial, real estate, and business matters on behalf of the principal (the person who signs the power of attorney). Sometimes the agent is called an "attorney in fact." The agent has the authority to act on the principal's behalf, but only to the extent the principal granted the power to act in the document. People who have Alzheimer's or Parkinson's generally should have a very broad, all-encompassing power of attorney.

Planning tip: Just having a durable power of attorney is not enough. Alzheimer's and Parkinson's patients should work with an elder law attorney to draft powers of attorney with these four key powers:

- The power to apply for public benefits (such as Medicaid) in case that is later needed for your care;
- The power to make unlimited gifts on your behalf and do Medicaid planning;
- The power to make decisions based on your overall well-being, not just from a financial perspective; and
- The power to create an irrevocable trust for you, and to remove or add assets to that trust.

In addition to signing a durable power of attorney with broad powers as described above, generally is it best for a person who has Alzheimer's or Parkinson's to make the power of attorney immediately effective. While many states allow "springing" powers of attorney that take effect only when the principal is determined to be unable to make his or her own decisions, that can cause problems. For example, as the disease progresses, the patient may be moving in and out of cognitive impairment, sometimes able to make decisions and sometimes not. That could complicate the use of the power of attorney. Moreover, some springing powers of attorney require that one or two physicians give their written opinion that the patient can no longer adequately make his or her own decisions. This process may sound like a good idea in theory. But in the real world, at best it adds undue complication during an already stressful time. At worst it creates ill-will and family fights and even leads to lawsuits when the family has to take a parent to a doctor but the parent, argumentative and unyielding due largely to his or her demented state, refuses to go.

Some people are reluctant to sign a power of attorney because they believe they are giving up their independence. That is not the case. Someone who signs a power of attorney continues to have the authority to act for themselves. In fact, they even retain the authority to cancel the power of attorney at any time, as long as they are mentally capable of doing so.

Another concern many people have about powers of attorney is that they worry the agent may mishandle their money, even take money for the agent's own use. This is always going to be a risk, but the agent will be held accountable by law to act only in your best interest. This is called a "fiduciary duty" and is imposed on your agent because of his or her position of trust. The agent must carefully track all receipts and expenses on your behalf. The court can require an agent to repay money that is lost through misconduct or gross negligence, and there are even criminal penalties involved for an agent who takes advantage of someone under a power of attorney.

Planning tip: An agent under a power of attorney always should keep careful records for financial dealings under a power of attorney. This includes keeping bank statements, cancelled checks, and expense receipts. Most importantly, always keep the principal's money separate from the agent's. Never combine or "co-mingle" accounts. The best way to do this is through separate checking accounts, and possibly using a credit card exclusively for the principal. Also, it is generally a good idea to maintain good communication among family members, which can avoid the resentment and disputes that often happen when other family members are not kept informed about the principal's finances.

§ 6.4.2. Managing Medical Matters: Health Care Powers of Attorney and Living Wills

One of the biggest worries for people who have Alzheimer's and Parkinson's is making sure that their families can make medical decisions if the disease robs them of the ability to make or communicate those decisions themselves. That's why it's so important to have a durable power of attorney for health care decisions. This document is sometimes called a "health care power of attorney," a "durable power of attorney for health care decisions," or a "health care proxy." It is a type of an advance medical directive, and it may include the authority of a "living will" (discussed below) for end of life decisions, or a separate living will document may be used in addition to the health care power of attorney.

A health care power of attorney is always a "springing" power of attorney. It only takes effect if you are unable to make or communicate your own decisions. However, like the durable power of attorney, the health care agent must act always in the principal's best interest and as directed by the document.

A health care power of attorney is more than just a living will. A living will is the earliest type of advance directive, and it directs whether or not to administer artificial life support if you become terminally ill and cannot state your own wishes. On the other hand, the health care power of attorney will allow your agent to make decisions other than for end of life. In addition, the health care power of attorney can give standards for care and also provide for organ donation or donation of your remains for research into the treatment of Alzheimer's or Parkinson's disease.

§ 6.4.3. Choosing Your Agents

Choosing your agent for the financial and health care powers of attorney bears careful thought. The agents under each document can be the same people, or you can choose different people. Typically, a family member acts as an agent but you may also select a trusted friend, or in some cases a lawyer or professional trust company. *Choose the person to serve as your agent based on who you think will do the best job for you, not based on your desire to be "fair" among your children.* The agent who deals with money must make sound financial decisions and be completely trustworthy in all financial dealings, preferably without his or her own financial worries. Ask yourself whether your agent, whether for financial or health care, will always act in your own best interests. And always be sure to talk with your agent so they know your wishes and how you would want them to act in certain situations. Particularly because Alzheimer's and Parkinson's tend to be long term illnesses and the power of attorney may need to be used for many years, your power of attorney should name back-up agents in case your primary agent is no longer available to act or dies. Otherwise, your power of attorney may become ineffective because no one remains who can serve as agent.

§ 6.4.4. Guardianship and Conservatorship

If a person who has Alzheimer's or Parkinson's reaches a stage where he or she can no longer make decisions for himself or herself, the court may need to get involved especially where there is no power of attorney in place. This should be avoided if possible. Guardianships and conservatorships can involve many thousands of dollars in attorney's fees, ongoing court costs, unnecessary delays, extra paper work, and family fights. And even if the Alzheimer's or Parkinson's patient intended to protect his or her life savings from the high costs of nursing home care, many states do not allow Medicaid planning though a guardianship or conservatorship. You should consult with an experienced elder law attorney in your state for the best course of action if a guardianship or conservatorship becomes necessary.

§ 6.5.
CARE FOR THE ALZHEIMER'S OR PARKINSON'S PATIENT

A care giving journey starts once the symptoms of Alzheimer's or Parkinson's become noticeable to others, and especially after the patient receives the diagnosis. This journey generally begins at home. Eventually the care needs may exceed the ability of the family to provide or pay for care at home, and then the person would move to assisted living or nursing home care.

§ 6.5.1. Being the Caregiver

Caring for a person who has Alzheimer's or Parkinson's disease means adapting over time. At first, only modest assistance may be needed. Later, more assistance will be needed. Perhaps clothes will need to be laid out, or the person will need help with dressing. You may prompt his or her memory by placing notes around the house. Eventually you may need to change door locks if your loved one tries to wander and turn down the water heater temperature in order to avoid burns. Care may progress to assistance with toileting, feeding, bathing, and making sure that the person does not fall and get injured, and even to full-time observation.

If you are the caregiver for a person who has Alzheimer's or Parkinson's, you should become familiar with the available respite care programs in your community. Designed to temporarily relieve family members, these programs provide a respite caregiver who comes into the house for a few hours, allowing you to go out, shop, see a movie, or just relax on your own. Taking care of yourself is the only way you can continue the care for your loved one.

Adult day care programs are another alternative for giving respite to caregivers. These programs provide socialization and therapeutic activities in a safe environment at a church or dedicated facility. While there is generally a charge, often the charge is reduced or even waived depending on financial circumstances.

The best way to start with getting help for being a caregiver at home, and accessing respite and adult day care programs, is to contact the local Area Agencies on Aging or the local chapter of the Alzheimer's or Parkinson's Associations. You may also find helpful suggestions from local nursing homes or other families who have had similar experiences.

§ 6.5.2. Paid Caregivers

Many people supplement the care at home with paid caregivers, or get all of the at-home care through paid caregivers. Medicare generally does not pay for home health care for custodial care, which is the type of care a person who has Alzheimer's or Parkinson's usually needs. Many states do have a Medicaid waiver program that lets people who need this care remain at home (and avoid the expense of a nursing home). This would require meeting the income and asset tests of your particular state for Medicaid qualification for these care at home programs. Many of these programs have long waiting lists that can delay participation.

Sometimes a family member may be paid to provide care for the person who has Alzheimer's or Parkinson's. In those situations, be sure to consult with an elder law attorney in your area, because there are tricky tax and Medicaid gifting issues that can trap the unwary.

§ 6.5.3. Hospice

Hospice care is a limited exception where Medicare can help pay for care at home. Hospice is designed for dying patients and requires that a doctor give an opinion that the patient will live only another six months or less. At that point the care changes from an attempt to cure the illness to comfort care. Because of the difficulties of determining when a person who has Alzheimer's or Parkinson's has reached the last stage of the disease, there are specific Medicare and National Hospice Organization guidelines for hospice care for non-cancer diseases including dementia and Parkinson's.

Planning tip: If you are providing care at home for a loved one, start exploring the possibility of hospice early. Talk with the doctor about this, and if the doctor balks or hesitates, consider talking with another doctor. Starting hospice doesn't mean you've given up. In fact, getting the additional help at home may be sufficient to overcome immediate health concerns, and the patient may even improve sufficiently to withdraw from hospice.

§ 6.5.4. Care at an Assisted Living Facility or Nursing Home

There are various options for care outside the home, which will depend upon the level of care needed for the person who has Alzheimer's or Parkinson's, the available care in the community, and the financial costs.

Assisted living facilities are often an appropriate choice for people who have Alzheimer's or Parkinson's when skilled nursing is not needed. This can be a good first move for the person who has the disease, as well as for the family caregivers who can no longer provide the care needed at home without ruining their own health.

When considering assisted living, pay close attention to how a person who has dementia will cope. Many people who have dementia become agitated and need a safe place to go outside their room. Look for a facility with at least one enclosed outdoor area like a courtyard and also a common space indoors where the resident can wander safely. In addition, look for facilities that offer a special care unit that is dedicated to residents who have dementia, even if not currently needed. These dedicated units will be more secure than a mixed setting, and the staff will be specially trained for working with people who have dementia and provide more extensive care and appropriate socialization.

Payment arrangements will vary by community. Many will charge monthly, without any long term commitment. Other communities will require an up front charge, and for communities that are part of a CCRC (Continuing Care Retirement Community) in particular, the up front charge can run into the tens or hundreds of thousands of dollars. Be sure to look for a community that meets your financial ability to pay, both now and in the future as care needs arise.

Sometimes an assisted living arrangement is desirable, but the family will be unable to pay all of the cost. In some states, there may be government benefits to assist with the cost of care, although generally Medicaid is reserved for nursing home care rather than assisted living. Veteran's benefits may also be available to help offset some of the costs of assisted living care. Most families pay for assisted living privately, either out of their own funds or through long term care insurance that was purchased previously when the resident was in good health.

The progression of the Alzheimer's or Parkinson's may require skilled nursing care at a nursing home. Making the decision to place a loved one in a nursing home is never easy. But when the care needs exceed the available care at home or in assisted living, or if Medicaid is needed to help cover the cost of care, then the nursing home is going to be the only option. However, not all nursing homes are equipped to handle residents who wander, and you may have special concerns over someone who is prone to falling. These will be important considerations as you select the nursing home.

Planning tip: For both assisted living and nursing home care, a care plan is developed when the resident arrives. Because of the special care needs for Alzheimer's and Parkinson's, be sure that the diagnosis is properly noted in the plan of care, and that there are activities appropriate for the resident's abilities. This care plan should be reviewed regularly, and updated when the resident's condition changes as the disease progresses.

§ 6.5.5. Getting Help Paying for Care

While outside the scope of this chapter, there are various ways to pay for the costs of care at home or in a care community. This can include private pay, long term care insurance, and Medicaid. Medicare does not help to pay for the cost of custodial care, but it can help pay for a brief time for rehabilitation in a skilled nursing home following a hospital stay.

Each state's rules will vary, but generally Medicaid planning can help protect the person who has Alzheimer's or Parkinson's and his or her family. Be sure to consider available veteran's benefits, including "aid and attendance" programs for a wartime veteran and the surviving spouse of a deceased wartime veteran.

It is critical to plan ahead to preserve family savings, preferably at least five years before paid care is needed if possible. Otherwise, once a person spends down to the point where Medicaid covers the cost of care, he or she must have next to no countable assets (often $2,000 or less) and then only gets to keep about $30 per month (not even a dollar per day!) from his or her Social Security check and pension. Proper planning often can set aside funds that allow the family to pay for extras not available when trying to live on the pittance allowed by Medicaid.

There are often special Medicaid rules that help to protect the spouse who remains at home, sometimes called the "community spouse."

Planning tip: *Be sure to start planning when you get the diagnosis of Alzheimer's or Parkinson's. Don't wait until the disease has taken its terrible toll.* If you wait, you will lose valuable years of planning time, and the disease may even rob you from being able to sign critical documents and take important planning steps to protect him yourself and your family. And, never get your Medicaid planning advice from the Medicaid office. They are under no obligation to tell you all of the available options to best protect yourself, your house, and your life savings. Instead, talk with an experienced elder law attorney who is familiar with the public benefits in your state.

§ 6.6.
CONCERNS ABOUT SAFE DRIVING
AND FINANCIAL MANAGEMENT

§ 6.6.1. Knowing What to Do About Driving

Alzheimer's and Parkinson's can impair a person to the point of not being safe to drive. As Parkinson's progresses, it can get more difficult to react quickly and to think of several things at once. Some people get blurry vision or begin seeing double. Drug therapy also may cause sleepiness, mental impairment, or even hallucinations. With Alzheimer's, deteriorating concentration, impaired judgment, and lack of memory all can result in disorientation, failure to understand traffic signals, and slow or poor driving decisions that endanger not only the driver but also others on the road. Studies have shown that a person who has Alzheimer's disease is twice as likely to be involved in a motor vehicle accident as a healthy driver of the same age. Studies also show that even mild Alzheimer's can pose risks, and the risks increase as the condition worsens.

Many people who have Alzheimer's and Parkinson's recognize a point when it is no longer safe to drive. However, others insist on driving when they should not. Family members and others should assess the situation and when necessary take away the keys. You should also contact your family member's physicians and share your concerns. Some persons will listen to the physician over their own family. Also, in some states the physician may forward a report to the state driving authorities, who can require that the person stop driving unless he or she passes a new driving test.

Planning tip: You should not transfer your parent's car into your own name if you have concerns about your parent continuing to drive. That's because a car owner is personally liable for an accident caused by someone else driving the car.

There are various strategies for preventing someone from driving. For some families it works well when the parent during the early stages of the disease signs a contract, agreeing to stop driving later when they may no longer be able to recognize the danger themselves. Sometimes it becomes necessary to hide keys or disable the car, or to remove the car altogether. If you disable the car, remember to discontinue the AAA membership too. And, if the car is removed, be sure to tell the police of the situation to avoid problems if the car is reported missing by your family member. And in all circumstances, you will need to develop an alternative plan for transportation so the person who has Alzheimer's or Parkinson's will not become isolated.

This is a difficult time, and family members need to approach this decision with compassion and love, but with a firm resolve to do what is needed to keep their loved one safe and to prevent injury to others.

§ 6.6.2. Managing Finances and Guarding Against Fraud

There are some concerns that ill-advised spending precedes actual detection of dementia that may be part of Alzheimer's and

Parkinson's. While making an occasional unnecessary purchase at the grocery store is not going to matter, this can become a very serious concern if the person buys big-ticket items or makes extremely risky investments that devastate the family finances. I have seen too many situations where the spouse and children have searched for how the ill spouse wasted money for years while his or her dementia worsened to the point that others started noticing, leaving the couple financially compromised.

In any case, it is clear that over time people who have dementias lose their ability to manage their own financial affairs. Usually the first signs are difficulties counting change, calculating a tip, or understanding the bank statement. You might start noticing new purchases on credit cards and unpaid and unopened bills lying around the house. This can be an early sign of Alzheimer's disease and dementia, and it can drain financial resources quickly.

Another major concern is increased vulnerability to being taken advantage of by strangers as well as by people known to the impaired person. Some types of fraud to watch for include the following:

- Home repair fraud, such as repairs to foundations, roofs, driveways, and trees;
- Dishonest door-to-door solicitations and scam charities;
- Long distance fraud through telephone, email, and mail;
- Credit card misuse and identity theft; and
- Abuse of a power of attorney by taking funds for personal use, or family members frightening the senior into giving up financial resources.

You may see indications that a person is being victimized, such as:

- Unexplained changes in bank balances and investments and/or large cash withdrawals;

- Payment overdue notices, unpaid utilities, and lapsed insurance policies; and
- Signs of physical or emotional abuse.

When and how to address these financial issues are just as difficult as dealing with safe driving issues, and often even more difficult. Proactive steps should be taken, which include planning in advance for delegating financial decision making through a power of attorney that names a trustworthy agent. In addition, moving money and investments into protected trust and banking arrangements can help. At a minimum, there should be increased supervision of finances to avoid the larger problems.

Another practical step to reduce the risk of fraud is to get an unlisted phone number. Also, you should reduce the amount of direct mail soliciting subscriptions and contributions, and perhaps use a service that will remove the senior's name from various "junk mail" lists. Make sure that someone is checking in with the senior on a regular basis by creating a care network that can include family members, neighbors, paid caregivers, lawn care service providers, house keepers, and even the postal delivery person and local fire fighters. If any new construction is seen at the house, someone should notify the family immediately.

It is also important that Social Security and other checks be direct-deposited as much as possible. A trusted family member can review finances and even help with paying bills through online computer banking. Even if the senior should no longer be in control of his or her own checkbook, this transition may be easier if the senior has a small amount of cash or a checkbook with a modest amount of cash in it. In some cases, the person may feel better with having voided checks on hand. The credit limit on credit cards should be reduced, or the cards cancelled altogether.

If an impaired senior reaches the point of endangering his or her own finances and future security due to cognitive impairment, action needs to be taken. If the senior is not willing to allow his or her family to help, or if there is no power of attorney in place and the senior lacks the capacity to sign one, or if the agent under the power of attorney is acting inappropriately, it may be necessary to begin a guardianship or conservatorship to protect the senior through court intervention.

If you suspect that someone is losing the capacity to manage his or her own financial affairs, pay close attention. This can be the first noticeable sign of dementia, indicating that the person may be losing the ability to live independently. Often the senior will be suspicious and resist efforts of help, regardless of earlier agreements and existing power of attorney arrangements. No matter what, it is critical to approach the transfer of financial authority with respect, compassion, and understanding.

For more information, visit the website of
The Elderlaw Firm at:
http://www.elderlawfirm.com.

[37] Alzheimer's Association, *2014 Alzheimer's Disease Facts and Figures*, available at http://www.alz. org/downloads/Facts_Figures_2014.pdf.

[38] Alzheimer's Association, *What Is Alzheimer's*, at http://www.alz.org/alzheimers_disease_what_is_ alzheimers.asp (last updated July 29, 2011).

[39] *Id.*

[40] *Id.*

[41] *Id.*

[42] *Id.*

[43] The Michael J. Fox Foundation for Parkinson's Research, *Parkinson's 101*, at http://www.mi-chaeljfox.org/living_aboutParkinsons_parkinsons101.cfm#q1 (last updated July 8, 2011).

[44] *Id.*

[45] *Id.*

[46] *Id.*

[47] *Id.*

[48] *Id.*

[49] National Parkinson Foundation, *Parkinson's Disease (PD) Overview*, at http://www.parkinson.org/ parkinson-s-disease.aspx (last visited Nov. 6, 2014).

[50] National Parkinson Foundation, *How is PD Treated?*, at http://www.parkinson.org/Parkinson-s-Disease/Treatment (last visited Nov.6, 2014).

CHAPTER 7

MEDICAID

Thorpe A. Facer, Esquire

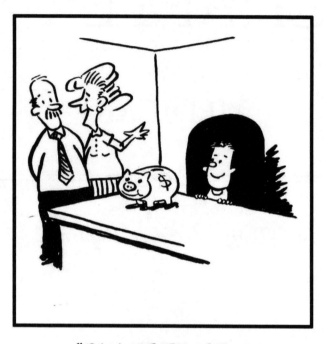

"CAN WE TRUST HIM
WITH OUR PIGGY BANK?"

"AN AGGRAVATED ASSAULT ON THE ENGLISH LANGUAGE, RESISTANT TO ATTEMPTS TO UNDERSTAND IT."

– The United States Supreme Court describing Medicaid law[51]

§ 7.1.
INTRODUCTION

Understanding Medicaid requires that we lay a little groundwork before we discuss details. In this chapter, we'll lay that groundwork, discuss the rules for qualifying for Medicaid, discuss important points to consider when planning for possible Medicaid issues in the future, and illustrate the various points with case studies to show how Medicaid works.

Four important points to remember that will help our discussion: First, Medicaid is a federal program funded by both the federal government and each state. The federal government sets forth guidelines which each state implements as it determines appropriate. The Medicaid rules are different in every state, and, while there are many similarities from state to state, there are important differences as well. For example, one state might count an individual retirement account (IRA) as an asset for qualification purposes while a neighboring state may not; if you live on the border between these two states, this difference in rules may make the difference between qualifying for Medicaid while retaining a sizeable asset (the IRA) or not qualifying at all.

Second, Medicaid is a needs based program; you have to meet asset and income limitations to qualify. We'll discuss those limitations in detail throughout this chapter. Because of the name similarity, confusing Medicaid with the Medicare program is easy to do. While a bit of an oversimplification, think of Medicare as health insurance that you "bought" by paying Medicare taxes while you worked, and in the case of Medicare Part B, that you continue to pay for through a deduction from your monthly social security benefits.

Think of Medicaid as nursing home insurance available only to those who meet asset and income limitations.

Third, Medicaid can have different names depending on what state you live in. Massachusetts calls its Medicaid program "MassHealth." California refers to its program as "Medi-Cal." And so forth. Some states have programs known as waiver programs that provide care under that state's Medicaid program to qualified recipients in their homes. Other states do not have waiver programs or their programs are poor and ineffectual.

Fourth, the figures used for determining Medicaid qualifications and exemptions vary state by state. The figures used in this chapter are as examples only. Not only do the figures vary state by state, but the figures change nearly every year. The Medicaid rules also change regularly. For these reasons, and as you will read over and over throughout this chapter, always consult a local and experienced elder law attorney when dealing with Medicaid issues.

7.2.
QUALIFICATION PROCESS

§ 7.2.1. Medical

You or a loved one needs Medicaid to pay for care whether in the home, in an assisted living-type facility, or, as is most common, in the nursing home. Let's talk about the qualification process that generally applies whether the care you seek is in the home, an assisted living facility, or the nursing home.

The threshold requirement of the qualification process is that you medically need the care. Many times, with the person who suffers from Alzheimer's disease or has had a stroke, the need for care is obvious. Nonetheless, the basic medical requirement is that you need help with some of the activities of daily living (ADLs) which are bathing, dressing, transferring from bed or chair, walking, eating, and using the toilet. Traditionally, for Medicaid to pay, you have to need help with any three of the six ADLs (a diagnosis of severe dementia or Alzheimer's is an automatic qualifier).

Once you are confirmed by your doctor as medically needing Medicaid to pay for your care, then you must meet income and asset limitations. These limitations vary for single or widowed persons and married couples. The limitations vary from state to state, but certain procedures are followed regardless.

§ 7.2.2. Assets

The first procedure in the qualification process is to divide assets into two categories: (1) exempt and (2) non-exempt or countable. Exempt assets do not count against you in the sense that owning these exempt assets does not affect your qualifying or not qualifying for Medicaid. Non-exempt or countable assets are considered by Medicaid in determining whether you qualify. Exempt assets are:

1. Your residence;
2. One motor vehicle of reasonable value although what is a reasonable value can vary from state to state;
3. Pre-paid or irrevocable funeral and burial plans (another area where requirements vary from state to state);

4. Cash value life insurance up to $1,500 of value for all policies combined, not per policy (the exact figure varies from state to state);

5. Normal household goods including personal jewelry; and

6. Other assets, most commonly $2,000 in cash, but the amount varies from a low of $999 in Missouri to a high of $13,800 in New York; for our purposes we'll use the figure of $2,000 throughout this chapter.

All other assets are countable with the caveat that some states exempt assets, such as an IRA, that generate income. The income is counted as part of evaluating the income limitations, but the asset is not. Similarly, some states exempt income producing real property such as rental houses or farmland. Check with your local elder law attorney for your state's rules.

Let's look at how the asset limitations would apply to a single or widowed person. John Smith owns his home, one car, and has $100,000 in the bank and in various investments. If John needs Medicaid to pay for his care, his assets will be evaluated as follows: His house and car will not be counted in determining his eligibility. His $100,000 in other assets will be. John will not qualify for Medicaid until the $100,000 is spent down leaving only $2,000. We'll discuss in the section on Medicaid Planning how best to accomplish the spend down.

Determining assets for a married couple is more complicated. In 1988, Congress passed a law commonly referred to as the Spousal Impoverishment Act. The purpose of this act was to avoid impoverishing the spouse who did not need Medicaid (the community spouse) while still qualifying the spouse who did need Medicaid (the nursing home spouse). As part of the Act, Congress set limits on the amount of countable assets the community spouse may keep as well as limits on income. These asset limits are called the Community Spouse Resource Allowance (CSRA).[52] These limits typically change each year, increasing in small amounts. For assets in 2011, the upper limit is $109,560 in countable assets while the lower limit is $21,912. While the upper limit figure is uniform in all states, the lower limit figure varies from state to state.

Most states divide the assets as follows. On what is called the snapshot date (the first day the Medicaid applicant is admitted to a health care facility for at least 30 continuous days and then applies for Medicaid benefits, but often the date the Medicaid application is filed is used instead), the married couple's countable assets are divided in two with each spouse being assigned one-half. If the one-half attributed to the community spouse is more than the lower limit ($21,912 typically) and less than the upper limit of $109,560, then the community spouse keeps all of those assets. The one-half of the assets assigned to the nursing home spouse will have to be spent down to $2,000 before he or she is eligible for Medicaid.

If the community spouse's one-half of the assets is less than the lower limit, then enough of the nursing home spouse's assets are assigned to the community spouse to bring his or her assets up to the lower limit. If the community spouse's one-half of the countable assets is greater than $109,560, then the excess is assigned to the nursing home spouse, the community spouse keeps the $109,560, and the nursing home spouse has to spend down the remainder. Here are some examples.

John and Jane Jones have $200,000 in countable assets on the snapshot date. Jane needs nursing home care and needs Medicaid to pay for it. The Medicaid caseworker will divide the $200,000 in countable assets in half, assigning $100,000 to Jane and $100,000 to

John who gets to keep his share of the assets. Jane has to spend down her $100,000 to $2,000 before she will qualify for Medicaid.

Now let's give John and Jane Jones $300,000 in countable assets. Again, the caseworker will divide the $300,000 in half, giving $150,000 to each. However, because John's share of $150,000 is higher than the allowed limit of $109,560, the difference of $40,440 is taken from him and reassigned to Jane who will now have to spend down her $150,000 plus the additional $40,440 taken from John before she qualifies for Medicaid. On the other end of the scale, if John and Jane only had $30,000 in countable assets, John would get to keep enough of Jane's one-half ($15,000) to bring his total up to the lower limit of $21,912. Jane would have to spend down the remaining $8,088 before Medicaid would pay for her care.

The process described above is what approximately two-thirds of the states do with regard to asset limitations for married couples. The other one-third of the states make this calculation differently. These states assign the first $109,560 to the community spouse. Any assets over the first $109,560 are assigned to the nursing home spouse and must be spent down to $2,000 to qualify for Medicaid. Repeating the first example above where John and Jane have $200,000 in countable assets, these states would assign John the first $109,560 and the remaining $90,440 would have to be spent down. Similarly, with $300,000 in assets, again the first $109,560 would be assigned to John while Jane would have to spend down $190,440. Finally, if John and Jane's total assets were only $30,000, then all $30,000 would be assigned to John, and Jane would not have to spend down any amount to qualify for Medicaid.

To summarize with respect to assets, the first step in evaluating assets is to divide them into exempt and countable assets. Exempt assets are not considered in determining whether a person qualifies for Medicaid. Only countable assets are used in determining eligibility. For single or widowed persons, the amount of countable assets you are allowed to have to qualify for Medicaid varies from state to state with the most common figure being $2,000. For married couples, the amount of countable assets the community spouse is allowed to keep also varies from state to state with the high being $109,560 and the typical low being $21,912. The nursing home spouse is only allowed the amount the single or widowed person can keep, $2,000 for discussion purposes. This sums up how assets are treated for Medicaid qualification purposes. Now let's turn to income qualification.

§ 7.2.3. Income

In the most basic sense, Medicaid treats income very simply. If you have enough income to pay your monthly care bill, you don't qualify for Medicaid. But, as always, the Medicaid rules make distinctions between single or widowed persons and married couples. A very few states make additional distinctions that make it even harder to qualify for Medicaid.

About sixteen of the states are what are called Income Cap states. In these states, if your income exceeds the "cap" figure set by the state, even if that income is insufficient to pay for your care bills, you do not qualify for Medicaid. All but one of the sixteen states set the cap limit at $2,022 (Oklahoma's cap is $3,000). In other words, if your income is $2,023 or more, but still insufficient to pay your monthly nursing home bill of $5,000, for example, you do not qualify for Medicaid. That's the bad news. The good news is that procedures have been worked out in the Income Cap states to divert income so as to reduce a person's income to below the cap thus allowing qualification for Medicaid. However, the procedures for doing this are beyond the scope of this chapter. Consult an experienced elder law attorney.

The remaining states only limit income in the sense that to qualify for Medicaid your income has to be insufficient to pay for your care. But what happens to your income if you do qualify for Medicaid? Again, the answer varies depending on whether you are single or widowed or married. Let's take the single person first.

For a single or widowed person, if your income is below the amount necessary to pay for your care, and you meet all the other requirements to qualify for Medicaid (medically necessary, asset limitations), then this is what happens to your income. First, you are allowed a personal needs allowance, the amount of which varies from state to state. The low is $30 per month while the high is $101.10 per month (Arizona). The average between all the states is about $50 per month, and we'll use that figure for discussion purposes throughout this chapter. Of your remaining income, you keep an amount equal to any health insurance or prescription drug plan premiums you pay. All the rest is paid to the nursing home as a co-pay. Here is an example for a single or widowed person.

Bill Green receives $3,000 per month in social security and pension income. He pays $150 per month in premiums for his Medicare supplement policy. Bill does not live in an income cap state. Nursing home care is his area is $5,500 per month. Because Bill's income is insufficient to pay for his nursing home care, he can qualify (provided he meets all the other requirements) for Medicaid to pay for his nursing home. What happens to his $3,000 in income? First, he is allowed to keep his personal needs allowance of $50. Then, he is allowed to continue paying for his Medicare supplement policy, so that $150 is also deducted. The remaining amount of his income,

$2,800, has to be paid to the nursing home each month as a co-pay for his care. Medicaid pays for the balance.

If, in this example with Bill having income of $3,000 per month, he lived in an income cap state, then he would see an experienced elder law attorney to learn how to divert part of his income so that he could otherwise qualify for Medicaid.

For married couples, once again, Medicaid treats income differently than for single or widowed persons. The Spousal Impoverishment Act previously mentioned not only protects community spouses from total loss of assets but it also protects the community spouse's income rights. But, as always, different states treat a married couple's income differently. Medicaid calls this income the Minimum Monthly Maintenance Needs Allowance (MMMNA) for the community spouse. The purpose of the MMMNA is to ensure that the community spouse has a minimum amount of income each month. Here's how it works.

About two-thirds of the states allow the community spouse to keep income within the range of $1,821 on the low end up to $2,739 on the high end. These states are called "range" states. The remaining states will allocate the maximum of $2,739 to the community spouse if that amount of income is available meaning that the married couple, between them, have income of at least $2,739. If their joint income is below that figure, the community spouse will get to keep it all but he or she is not entitled to more to bring it up to the maximum of $2,739.

For example, Greg Williams has monthly income of $900. His wife, Susan Williams, has monthly income of $1,989. Susan has to go into the nursing home and have Medicaid pay for her care. What happens to her income? If Greg and Susan live in a "range" state, then Greg will be allowed to keep enough of Susan's income to increase his monthly income up to the low end of the income range, typically $1,821. This means he will keep $921 of Susan's income as his own. Of Susan's remaining income, she will be allocated her personal needs allowance and whatever amount she pays in premiums for health insurance or a prescription drug plan, and the rest will go as a co-pay to the nursing home.

In a non-range state, a state where Greg is allowed to supplement his income with his wife's income up to $2,739, he would be allowed to keep $1,839 of Susan's monthly income as his own. Obviously, this is a much better result from Greg's point of view than if he lived in a range state. If Greg did live in a range state, and his income was somewhere within the allowable range, then he would keep all his income but not be allowed to supplement it with any of Susan's income. In a range state, so long as your income falls anywhere within the range, that's what you keep. You cannot supplement your income up to the high end of the range.

What if Greg's income is more than the maximum of $2,739, then what happens? From a practical standpoint, he gets to keep all of his income while all of Susan's income, minus her personal needs allowance and any insurance premiums, is used as a co-pay to the nursing home. For example, if Greg's income is $4,000 per month, he is not entitled to any of Susan's income since his income is already greater than the maximum of $2,739, but he does get to keep all of his $4,000 of income and doesn't have to help pay for any of Susan's nursing home care. However, this is not the case in New York and, depending on current trends, may not be the case much longer in other states. Federal law allows states to require Greg to use up to 25% of his excess income to help pay for Susan's care. In our example of Greg having monthly income of $4,000, the law would allow a state to require Greg to pay $315.25 (25% of his income in excess of

$2,739) to the nursing home for Susan's care. To date, only New York is actively pursuing this 25% of the excess income.

To summarize how Medicaid treats income, your income must be less than the monthly cost of your care to qualify for Medicaid in a non-income cap state. In an income cap state, if your income exceeds the cap ($2,022 per month), then you do not qualify although there are legal procedures to solve this problem. Of your income, you are allowed to keep a personal needs allowance (around $50 per month) and an amount necessary to pay health insurance or prescription drug plan premiums, and the rest is used as a co-pay to the nursing home or other facility. For married couples, the community spouse is allowed to keep his or her own income, and if that income falls below a certain range ($1,821 to $2,739), the community spouse can supplement his or her income with income drawn from the nursing home spouse.

To this point, we have been concerned with the qualification process for single persons and married couples. Let's look at several case studies to illustrate how this would work.

§ 7.2.4. Case Studies

CASE STUDY #1: Jim and Ruth Smith have been married for fifty years. Jim was diagnosed with Alzheimer's disease a year before. For most of that year, Ruth has been able to care for Jim at home, but a week ago, while Ruth was doing the grocery shopping, Jim wandered away from their house. He was found blocks away, mumbling incoherently to himself. He needs nursing home care immediately. Ruth and Jim's assets are as follows:

Savings account................$55,000
CDs............................$85,000

Money market account.….....$17,000

Checking account.…..…....$3,000

Residence (no mortgage).….$80,000

Jim gets a social security check for $1,800 each month; Ruth's check is $900. Her eyes fill with tears as she says, "At $5,500 to the nursing home every month, our entire life savings will be gone in less than two years!" What's more, she's afraid she won't be able to pay her monthly bills because a neighbor told her that the nursing home will be entitled to all of Jim's social security check. When Jim applies to Medicaid for help paying the nursing home, how will the caseworker handle their assets and income?

First, the caseworker will divide their assets into countable and non-countable or exempt assets. Of the assets listed above, the house is exempt and not counted in determining eligibility. The remaining assets total $160,000. If Jim and Ruth live in a range state, Ruth will be allowed to keep one-half of those assets, $80,000, as her own. Jim will be assigned the remaining $80,000 in assets which he will have to spend down to $2,000 before he qualifies for Medicaid. If Ruth and Jim live in a non-range state, Ruth will be allowed to keep the first $109,560 of their countable assets. The remainder will have to be spent down by Jim to $2,000.

In a range state, since Ruth's income of $900 is well below the minimum allowed to a community spouse, she will be able to "take" enough of Jim's income of $1,800 to increase her monthly income to the minimum of $1,821. If she lived in a non-range state, then Ruth would be entitled to take all of Jim's income of $1,800 to supplement her monthly income because their combined income is still below the figure of $2,739 allowed the community spouse in a non-range state. To determine if you live in a range or non-range state, consult your local elder law attorney.

What is the end result for Ruth and Jim? Jim's nursing home care will be paid for but Ruth will be left with diminished assets and income that is, in a range state, only two-thirds of what they had before Jim entered the nursing home. While this is a better result than the total impoverishment Ruth feared, it still leaves her struggling to make ends meet. Advance planning, which will be discussed briefly near the end of this chapter, could have provided a much better outcome for Ruth and Jim.

CASE STUDY #2: Ralph Jones needs nursing home care. He is a widower living alone in his home. One week ago, he fell and broke his hip. After surgery and a short stay in the hospital, he is being discharged to a nursing home. His adult children are being told by the social worker that Ralph can no longer live on his own, that he needs to be in a nursing home for the rest of his life. Ralph's assets are:

> Savings account................$5,000
> CDs............................$15,000
> Money market account........$22,000
> Checking account............$3,000
> Residence (no mortgage).....$60,000

Ralph's income consists of social security of $1,240 per month and a small pension of $82 per month. He pays a premium for a Medicare supplement policy of $130 per month. Can Ralph qualify for Medicaid and, if so, how?

As before, the first step is to classify Ralph's assets as either countable or exempt. Of the assets listed above, his house is exempt. Ralph's countable assets total $45,000. To qualify for Medicaid,

Ralph will have to spend $43,000 of his assets, leaving him just the $2,000 allowed by Medicaid.

Ralph's income is treated similarly. Of his total income of $1,322, he will be allowed to keep his small personal needs allowance and the money to pay his insurance premium of $130, but the rest will have to be paid to the nursing home. Ralph's children are distraught at this news because they know that Ralph will need extra items that the personal needs allowance won't pay for such as dentures, eyeglasses, hearing aids, clothes, toiletries, a phone in his room; the list goes on and on. The adult children will have to pay for those items out of their own pockets or Ralph will have to go without. Advance planning for Ralph could have greatly improved his financial situation and the quality of his life.

§ 7.3.
MEDICAID APPLICATION ISSUES

What could be easier? Go down to your local Medicaid office, pick up and fill out an application, turn it in, and you're qualified. Not exactly. While we have discussed medical, asset, and income qualification issues, other aspects come into play when a caseworker evaluates your application. This section will discuss some of those issues.

§ 7.3.1. Understanding the Application

Medicaid applications vary in length and complexity from state to state. A detailed discussion of each state's application is beyond the scope of this chapter. The intent here is to simply highlight a few common issues and emphasize the need to understand exactly what the application is asking and how the caseworker will evaluate your answers.

"Do you intend to return to your home?" Eight simple words that we all understand. But answering that question incorrectly can convert the home from an exempt asset that does not count against the applicant into a countable asset that will need to be sold and the money spent on nursing home and medical care. Why?

The house of a Medicaid applicant only retains its exempt status if the person intends to return to the home. But let's be honest. Unless a person is discharged to a nursing home to receive a short period of therapy and rehabilitation, such as learning to walk again after a knee replacement (in which case Medicaid is not involved in paying for the care), that person is not likely to come out of the nursing home. In other words, the applicant knows, the family knows, and the caseworker knows, that the person is not likely ever to return home. Nonetheless, the question needs to be answered with a "yes" or the home loses its exempt status.

One more example. As discussed in case study #1 above, in the case of a married couple, if the community spouse's income is too low, he or she is eligible to have some or all of the nursing home spouse's income assigned to her to supplement her own income. But if the married couple did not know of this benefit and did not properly ask for it on the application, they may not be told about it, and the community spouse would lose income he or she was otherwise entitled to receive.

§ 7.3.2. Timing, Look-back, and Gifting Issues

When to file the Medicaid application can be a difficult issue as well due to the convoluted Medicaid laws and regulations. Complicating this matter further is a law known as the Deficit Reduction Act of 2005 (DRA). This federal bill was signed into law on February 8, 2006. Ninety percent of the states have adopted the regulations required by this bill. The other 10% are in varying stages of adopting the new rules. Further complicating understanding the Medicaid rules state-by-state is that, while the DRA became effective on February 8, 2006, different states have adopted its regulations at different times with different effective dates. These different effective dates highlight yet again the need to consult an experienced elder law attorney in your state.

The DRA changed many rules for qualifying for Medicaid. The two most commonly discussed are the look-back period and the calculation of the penalty period. The look-back period is the time frame during which Medicaid can "look back" at your finances to ensure that you meet all the rules for qualifying for Medicaid. The look-back period is not a period of disqualification or penalty; it is nothing more than the length of time for which Medicaid can require you to provide your financial information. For example, if the lookback period is five years, and you apply on January 1, 2011, then Medicaid can require you to provide complete financial records and disclosure for the five years prior to your application. Before the DRA, look-back periods were three years except for some trusts which had a look-back period of five years. After the DRA, look-back periods are five years long.

Penalty periods are time frames, expressed in terms of months, during which a Medicaid applicant is not eligible for Medicaid to pay for his or her nursing home expenses. Penalty periods are assessed when an applicant violates a Medicaid rule, usually by making an uncompensated transfer (gift) of some sort. Regardless of whether a state has adopted the DRA, the length of penalty periods is calculated the same way (more on that in a moment). But calculating the date the penalty period starts has changed. Before the DRA, the penalty period started on the first day of the month in which you made the gift. Post-DRA, the penalty period does not start until the applicant is in the nursing home and is otherwise qualified for Medicaid (meaning he has spent down all of his assets except for the amount allowed to be kept). Let's look at a couple of examples.

§ 7.3.3. DRA Case Studies

CASE STUDY BEFORE ADOPTION OF THE DRA: On February 1, 2008, Grandma Jones gives her grandson $50,000 to help pay for his college expenses. The average cost of a month in the nursing home where Grandma Jones lives is $5,000. Taking the amount of the gift ($50,000) and dividing it by the cost of one month of care ($5,000) you get the number ten. This number ten represents the number of months Grandma Jones is penalized for making the $50,000 gift. And remember that the penalty means that for ten months, Medicaid won't pay for Grandma Jones' care in the nursing home. However, this penalty period started on February 1, 2008, and expired ten months later. If Grandma Jones didn't need nursing home care until December 2008 or after, her penalty period would have expired and would not be a factor in deciding when her application should be filed. Unfortunately, this is not true under the DRA.

CASE STUDY AFTER ADOPTION OF THE DRA: Same scenario: Grandma Jones gives $50,000 as a gift to her grandson. The monthly cost of nursing home care is $5,000. The calculation of the length of the penalty period is the same: Divide the amount of the gift ($50,000) by the monthly cost ($5,000) and you get the same figure of a ten month penalty. Calculating when the penalty starts, however, is where everything changes for the worse for Grandma Jones under the DRA.

Now Grandma Jones' penalty does not start until she is in the nursing home and has spent her countable assets down to $2,000. If she needed nursing home care in January 2013, four years and eleven months after the gift, and her Medicaid application was filed, she would be assessed a ten month penalty that started then. Who would pay for her care during these ten months? Most states have programs whereby an applicant can ask that the penalty period be waived, but few states grant hardship waivers. End result for Grandma Jones: She faces a ten month period during which her nursing home care will not be paid unless she has family who can afford to help.

Grandma Jones' predicament illustrates why the timing of filing a Medicaid application is so important. If her application had not been placed on file until five years and one day after the gift was made, she would have faced no penalty at all. Knowing the rules and waiting an extra few weeks to file the Medicaid application would have saved Grandma Jones much worry and her family nearly $50,000.

Gifting issues are trickier. Not a month goes by that someone doesn't ask, "I've heard I can give away $13,000 per year without tax consequences. Is this true?" The question is a good one but is fundamentally flawed because it confuses Medicaid law with federal gift tax law, which does allow a person to gift up to $13,000 per year per recipient without paying federal gift taxes. Medicaid can't prevent someone from making a gift in accordance with federal law, but it will penalize the gift if it falls within the applicable look-back period. So, what federal gift tax law allows, Medicaid law penalizes. Applying for veteran's benefits further complicates this situation. If you are a veteran or the spouse of a veteran, make sure to read the chapter on veteran's benefits.

Making a penalized transfer can be done without realizing it. A common example is the widow who puts an adult child on the deed to her house. If the house is worth $100,000, and the widow puts her adult son on the deed, she has just made a $50,000 gift that Medicaid will penalize. Forgiving a debt, such as a loan to a child, can also be a gift. If the person lives in a state that has not yet adopted the DRA, there may not be a problem because the penalty period may have expired before the need for Medicaid. If the person lives in a state that has adopted the DRA, then the timing of the filing of the Medicaid application will be critical.

§ 7.3.4. Application Information

Your elder law attorney will have a complete list of information that your state requires to be submitted with the Medicaid application. At a minimum, an applicant has to provide proof of citizenship; marital status; death certificate for deceased spouse; a photo ID; copies of social security, Medicare, and health insurance cards; information on any pre-paid funeral or burial plans; and complete and comprehensive financial information for the entire look-back period. This information includes all open or closed bank accounts, all investments, life insurance policies, income information, annuities, and literally everything to do with your finances that occurred during the look-back period.

People sometimes ask, "How does Medicaid find out about my finances?" The answer is simple: you have to tell them. Failing to do so or hiding assets or income are violations of federal law and, when discovered, will be penalized. That means fines and possible time in jail. No applicant for Medicaid should do anything other than make full and proper disclosure of all required information.

§ 7.4.
MEDICAID AND ESTATE PLANNING

§ 7.4.1. Medicaid Planning

Medicaid planning is the art and science of working within the Medicaid laws and rules to preserve assets to improve the quality of life of the person receiving Medicaid benefits, the quality of life of that person's spouse, and to improve the quality of life of the person's loved ones. Medicaid planning is analogous to tax planning. Tax planning does not seek to evade paying taxes, it only seeks to minimize the amount of taxes owed through good pre-planning and taking advantage of the rules in the Internal Revenue Code. Medicaid planning works the same way.

Why do Medicaid planning? A true story illustrates one reason. Two adult daughters visited their mother in the Alzheimer's unit of the local nursing home. This lovely elderly lady, who needs Medicaid to pay for her care, has hearing aids, the kind that are small and fit inside the ear. While the two daughters talked to her, the mother's hearing aid fell out. Mom picked it up and held it in the palm of her hand for a moment, looking at it. Her daughters thought she was about to insert it back into her ear. Instead, with a quick movement, the mother popped the hearing aid into her mouth and started to chew. She thought it was a piece of candy! She chewed the hearing aid hard enough to destroy it, to crack the hearing aid's battery case, and to chip and damage several teeth.

Who pays to replace the hearing aid? Who pays to repair her teeth? In many states, Medicaid will not pay for such things. Medicaid doesn't pay for eyeglasses in many states or pays so rarely (one pair of glasses every five years) that it's tantamount to not paying at all. Medicaid does not pay for clothes. If the Medicaid recipient wants a phone in her room, she pays for it herself. If she wants a television in her room, she pays. What Medicaid does allow her to have is a personal needs allowance so small that it more tantalizes by what it cannot pay than for what it does pay. Medicaid planning sets funds aside to be used for the benefit of the person needing help. Medicaid planning improves the quality of the person's life.

§ 7.4.2. Estate Planning

Estate planning is discussed in other chapters of this book. What needs to be remembered for Medicaid purposes is that people sometimes "die in the wrong order." Reasonably enough, most of us think of the spouse in the nursing home as most likely to die first. He wouldn't be in the nursing home if he wasn't sick or disabled. We think the community spouse will outlive the nursing home spouse, but it doesn't always happen that way.

Most married couples have what are commonly referred to as reciprocal wills. These wills say all to wife if husband dies first and all to husband if wife dies first, and when both are gone, then to the children. What if the husband is in the nursing home on Medicaid and the wife is healthier and in the home? They have reciprocal wills. And then the wife dies first. Who inherits with reciprocal wills? The husband does. What does Medicaid do? It stops paying for the husband's nursing home care until he has exhausted the money inherited from his wife. Remember that the wife, as the community spouse, was able to keep half of their assets up to $109,560 plus the exempt assets such as the house and the car. Now the husband in the nursing home owns all those assets, and they will have to be spent down to nothing before he again qualifies for Medicaid to pay for his care.

This unexpected and potentially devastating result could have—and should have—been avoided with the use of bypass planning. This planning would have set up the couple's estate planning documents to avoid this result, allowing the nursing home husband to remain qualified for Medicaid while safeguarding the other assets. See the chapter on estate planning for more details.

§ 7.4.3. Spend Down Strategies

The spend down is the amount of countable assets a person has to spend before qualifying for Medicaid. Accomplishing this spend down to best benefit the Medicaid applicant and the family is an important part of understanding Medicaid planning. Key to understanding the spend down is differentiating between compensated and uncompensated transfers.

A compensated transfer is just what it sounds like: you get something of fair market value for your money. For example, you buy a car for $20,000; assuming the car is worth $20,000, that's a compensated transfer. An uncompensated transfer is a gift from you to someone else. You sell your $20,000 car to one of your children for $100. That's an uncompensated transfer of $19,900 and a compensated transfer of $100. Under Medicaid law, compensated transfers are allowed; uncompensated transfers may be penalized.

If a married couple has $100,000 that has to be spent down because one of them needs nursing home care, what's the best way to accomplish that spend down? A detailed answer would be specific to that couple's exact circumstances, but general ideas for spend down might include fixing up the house (particularly with older couples, major repairs are often postponed because of worry over how to pay for care; now is the time to make those repairs), buying a better car for the community spouse, paying off debt, pre-paying funerals, and so forth. If the community spouse's income is low, using some of the spend down to purchase a Medicaid compliant annuity might be a good choice as a way to convert a countable asset—cash—into an income stream for the community spouse. Re-titling ownership of assets might make sense, and checking designated beneficiaries is a must in all situations to make sure someone on Medicaid does not receive money from life insurance policies, an IRA, or other similar assets. All these strategies are dependent on an applicant's specific circumstances.

Something to remember: once the Medicaid application has been filed, the only allowable compensated transfers to accomplish the spend down are to pay medical and related bills such as for care in the nursing home. Once the application is filed, you lose all flexibility in accomplishing the spend down.

§ 7.4.4. Powers of Attorney

This is a subject that is covered in other chapters of this book. The point here, vis-à-vis Medicaid issues, is that powers of attorney have to be drawn to allow the agent the right and authority to do the planning necessary to preserve assets in the event of incapacity of the principal. Too many standard forms do not include these kinds of powers.

§ 7.4.5. Estate Recovery

A final reason to do Medicaid planning is to protect your house. We Americans love our homes; we take pride in home ownership. Medicaid threatens aspects of that ownership.

A common myth is that Medicaid will take your house when you apply. Like many myths, there is a sliver of truth behind the statement. Medicaid will not take your house when you apply. However, if that house is owned by you, the Medicaid applicant, when you die, Medicaid will place a lien on the property for the amount of benefits paid on your behalf. If Medicaid paid, for example, $50,000 for your care while you were alive, after you're gone, a $50,000 lien will be placed on the property.

Some states are aggressive about pursuing that lien and require that the house be sold as soon as possible to pay it off. Other states sit back and wait for the property to be sold, knowing that when the sale closes, the lien will have to be paid off and the state will recover its funds. Safe to say that, as more states suffer budget crises, aggressively pursuing liens will become more common.

Several strategies exist for preserving the house. These include very limited situations when the house can be gifted without penalty to an adult child, a handicapped child, or a sibling. Pre-planning strategy may use irrevocable trusts to save the house and other property. All spend down strategies require a thorough and comprehensive knowledge of Medicaid, trust, tax, and other laws.

§ 7.5.
CONCLUSION

Medicaid is a complicated system of federal and state rules, with each state writing their own rules and regulations. Lengthy books have been written on Medicaid, taking three hundred pages to discuss what this chapter does in twenty or so. What is the answer? Consult your experienced, local elder law attorney on any issue involving Medicaid, from pre-planning to estate planning to Medicaid planning to Medicaid crisis planning to application filing issues. Any situation involving Medicaid demands the specialized knowledge of an elder law attorney.

For more information, visit the website of
Facer Law Office at:
www.facerlawoffice.com.

[51] *Schweiker v. Gray Panthers*, 453 U.S. 34, 43 (1981).

[52] Another frustration in understanding the Medicaid rules is that each state is free to name a concept, such as the Community Spouse Resource Allowance, whatever it chooses. For example, in Illinois the CSRA is called the Community Spouse Asset Allowance (CSAA). Check with your local elder law attorney regarding your state's terminology.

CHAPTER 8

SPECIAL MONTHLY PENSION AVAILABLE THROUGH THE VETERANS ADMINISTRATION

Michael L. Brumbaugh, Esquire

Accredited Attorney by the Veterans Administration

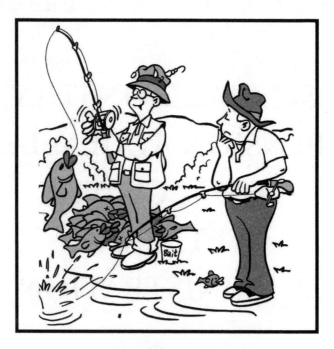

"THERE ARE LOTS OF
DECISIONS WE NEED TO MAKE...
YOU BETTER WATCH OUT
FOR THE BAITED HOOK."

There is a wonderful, almost secret, benefit available only to certain veterans who served during a period of war or conflict. This benefit is also extended to the spouses and widows of such veterans. Unfortunately, very few of those qualified for the benefit know it exists. Even fewer actually know how it works. Further adding to the secrecy and confusion of the benefit are the various names used to refer to it, such as "non-service connected disability pension," "non-service connected pension," "veterans pension program," "special monthly pension," "improved pension," "special pension," "VA pension," and "aid and attendance."

For purposes of clarity, we will refer to the benefit as a "Special Monthly Pension." Below, we will describe the source of the benefit and what the benefit entails, distinguish it from Disability Compensation, describe the basic criteria that must be met in order to qualify for the benefit, and provide some examples of how the benefit might apply. Finally, we will discuss some of the planning opportunities that are available, as well as some "planning techniques" to be wary of that might leave you worse off than doing nothing.

Before we go much further though, we would like to thank all the veterans for their service and for the sacrifices they and their families have made. For those of us who have never served, we can only imagine the hardships you have endured. Without your service, we would not enjoy our many freedoms and liberties that we too often take for granted.

The Special Monthly Pension is one of many benefits and programs offered and administered through the Veterans Administration (also referred to herein as "VA"). These benefits and programs offer much help and assistance to veterans. However, partially due to there being so many benefits and programs, it is often difficult to find someone at the VA who is knowledgeable about the Special

Monthly Pension program. In fact, trying to find someone who has meaningful knowledge about the benefit can feel like the proverbial hunt for the needle in the haystack. This often creates the second roadblock people run into when trying to learn more about this benefit. (The first roadblock is the fact that most people potentially eligible for the program do not even know it exists.) The problem occurs when someone who has heard about the program calls the VA and seeks information about the program. It is not uncommon for the person calling to be told the benefit does not exist (often because the caller referred to the benefit by a different name, and sometimes just because the VA employee is not familiar with the program).

If the VA employee is familiar with the benefit, the employee will often ask the caller a couple of questions about their income and assets and will quite often tell the caller he or she does not qualify for the benefit. This answer is often wrong or incomplete. One example of this is in a case where the income has been spent on out of pocket health expenses – expenses that the VA employee didn't ask about. The caller does not immediately qualify, but easily could if he or she worked with an elder law attorney to create a plan to obtain the benefit.

The volume of incorrect and incomplete answers that the VA provides to callers led to an article that highlighted the amount of incorrect information callers received about VA benefits. The article, by Chris Adams of Knight Ridder Newspapers,[53] used mystery callers to call the Department of Veterans Affairs. Twenty-two percent (22%) of the answers the callers received were completely wrong, twenty-three percent (23%) of the answers were "minimally correct," and twenty percent (20%) of the answers were "partially correct." Nineteen percent (19%) of the answers were "completely correct" and sixteen percent (16%) were "mostly correct."

Although the VA indicated in the article that steps would be put in place to provide more accurate information to callers, our own clients still tell us about mistaken information they receive from the VA. It is not unusual for them to be told the Special Monthly Pension benefit does not even exist!

You are probably asking, "So exactly what is the Special Monthly Pension?" This is a benefit provided only to a certain class of veterans (and their spouses/widows). The U.S. government has recognized that the men and women who served during periods of war or conflict have made special sacrifices; the Special Monthly Pension was created for those veterans and their widows.

The benefit is needs-based and helps eligible veterans or their widows who need financial assistance due to limited assets and incomes. It helps those whose incomes have been used to pay for out of pocket expenses incurred due to poor health, illness, or disability.

For those who qualify, the VA pays up to about $2,000.00 per month. In order to qualify, the veteran must be disabled and meet certain income and asset requirements. At its core, the benefit is a special thank-you program for veterans who served during a time of war or conflict who now need some extra help. Before we dig deeper into the requirements, let's distinguish the Special Monthly Pension from a much better known VA benefit – Disability Compensation.

Almost all veterans are familiar with the Disability Compensation benefit, even if they do not know it by name. The Disability Compensation benefit is different than the Special Monthly Pension in almost every important detail. In order to qualify for the Disability Compensation benefit, the veteran must show that he or she has an illness or injury that occurred during the veteran's service or that occurred after service, but was caused by something the veteran experienced during service. Appropriate examples include a veteran who loses a limb while serving or gets diabetes as a result of Agent Orange exposure.

For the Disability Compensation benefit, the VA will give the veteran a percentage disability rating based upon the degree the person is injured. The veteran then receives a monthly benefit, the size of which is determined by the disability rating. The greater the disability, the higher the rating; therefore, the more compensation the veteran will receive. For the Disability Compensation benefit, unlike the Special Monthly Pension, the veteran must be able to prove that the illness or injury is the result of his or her service.

There are other notable qualification differences between the Disability Compensation program and the Special Monthly Pension benefit. For the Disability Compensation Program, there is no need for the veteran to have served during a period of war or conflict. Also, the veteran can qualify for the Disability Compensation benefit regardless of his or her income or how much he or she has in assets.

The Special Monthly Pension program looks at whether the Veteran (or his or her spouse or widow) is disabled, but the program does not require the disability to have been caused in service. In fact, most of the clients we assist are not disabled from their service, but instead are disabled from illness or disease, such as Parkinson's, MS, Lou Gehrig's, Alzheimer's, strokes, heart attacks, or other sources.

The Special Monthly Pension program has a rather odd and far reaching definition of disability. First, if you are over age 65 and . . . actually, that is enough by itself! The government says that for the purposes of the Special Monthly Pension, if you are over 65 years of age, you will be treated as if you are "disabled." So even if you are fit as a fiddle and golf four times a week, if you are over 65, you meet the disability component of the Special Monthly Pension. However, if you are over 65 and fit as a fiddle, don't get too excited about the Special Monthly Pension, as you probably won't meet the other elements needed to qualify.

Most of the individuals we help meet the disability element because they are over age 65. If the veteran is younger than 65, the veteran must be permanently and totally disabled through no willful misconduct of his or her own.

The next element that must be met is the requirement that the veteran serve during a period of war or conflict. The government has set the wartime and conflict periods as follows:

Mexican Border:	May 9, 1916 to April 5, 1917
World War I:	April 6, 1917 to November 11, 1918 April 1, 1920 if served in Russia
World War II:	December 7, 1941 to December 31, 1946
Korean War:	June 27, 1950 to January 31, 1955
Vietnam War:	For a veteran who served in Vietnam: February 28, 1961 to May 7, 1975 For all other veterans: August 5, 1964 to May 7, 1975
Persian Gulf War:	August 2, 1990 to [date not yet determined]

In order to meet the service during war or conflict requirement, the veteran must have served in active duty for at least 90 consecutive days and at least one of those days of service had to fall within the above wartime/conflict periods. Additionally, the veteran cannot have been dishonorably discharged.

The next element is the asset limitation. If the veteran has too much in the way of assets, the veteran will not qualify for the Special Monthly Pension. When looking at assets, the VA considers all the assets of the household, but they exclude the residence itself, the typical household contents (investment quality art and antiques might cause a problem), and the family car. All other assets are counted (we will call these assets "countable assets"). Countable assets include cash, checking accounts, savings accounts, CDs, IRAs, stocks, bonds, etc.

How much are you allowed to have? While this is an excellent question, the answer is not as easy as you might expect. You may have heard that a single person or a married couple can have $80,000.00 of countable assets. This is an oft-mentioned figure, but it is better to think of this figure as a loose rule of thumb. The VA's regulations do not provide an exact dollar amount. Instead, the regulations provide a rather vague standard, which ultimately leads to a subjective decision by the person at the VA processing the claim. The rules state the VA will look at the assets, life expectancy, and needs of the veteran to determine if he or she qualifies. Thus, even on something that you would think would be simple, such as how much assets can be kept, the government makes the determination somewhat difficult.

Another qualification is a limitation on the amount of income you can receive. Again, the Special Monthly Pension rules make this more complicated than you would expect. Instead of simply looking at net income, the VA has come up with its own unique way to assess income known as Income for Veterans Administration Purposes, often referred to as "IVAP."

To determine your IVAP, the VA counts your *gross* household income from all sources. This includes your Social Security, pension, and other sources of income such as dividends and interest. Once the gross household income is determined, all non-reimbursed health related expenses are subtracted. This includes nursing home expenses, assisted living costs, out-of-pocket doctor bills and prescription costs, and health insurance premiums. If the person still lives at home, he or she cannot subtract regular household expenses such as mortgage or rent payments, property taxes, household insurance, utilities, and food. However, deductions for home health care agency expenses are allowed.

To determine IVAP, subtract the non-reimbursed health related expenses from the gross household income. Now that we have IVAP, what do we do with it? IVAP is important because the VA takes the IVAP figure and compares it to the maximum Special Monthly Pension the veteran is eligible to receive. If the IVAP is less than the maximum Special Monthly Pension amount, the veteran will receive some amount of pension. If the IVAP is more than the maximum amount, then the veteran will not receive a Special Monthly Pension. There are various categories of Special Monthly Pension, which will be discussed below.

Please remember that if you are 65 years of age and healthy, the Special Monthly Pension rules say you are disabled enough to receive the benefit. So, if you meet all of the other requirements and are 65, you will be eligible to receive some amount of Special Pension (so long as your IVAP is less than the Special Monthly Pension amount). Someone that has very limited income will get the lowest rate.

The next lowest rate is for "housebound" veterans, also considered the lowest level of disability. A veteran is considered housebound if he or she is substantially confined to his or her residence due to a disability that is likely to remain through his or her lifetime.

The highest level of disability is the "Aid and Attendance" level. To get this Special Monthly Pension amount, the veteran must show that he or she is in a nursing home, blind or nearly blind, or in need of regular aid to perform the basic activities of daily living. Activities of daily living, often called "ADLs," include bathing, dressing, toileting, and eating.

The veteran *or* the veteran's spouse can meet the disability requirement. The Special Monthly Pension is available not only to a veteran or a veteran who has a disabled spouse, but also to a veteran's widow/widower. A higher amount is paid to a veteran with a spouse, a lower amount to a single veteran and the lowest amount to the widow/widower of a veteran. However, that approximate $1,000.00 per month might make all the difference as to whether the widow/widower can afford to pay for care at home or in an assisted living facility, instead of going to a nursing home.

Another nice thing about the Special Monthly Pension is that it is tax-free. If you had to invest money to generate $2,000.00 per month, you would have to have more than half a million dollars. In fact, $500,000.00 receiving five percent (5%), would provide $25,000 per year before taxes.

THE SPECIAL MONTHLY PENSION RATES AS OF THE BEGINNING OF 2012 ARE AS FOLLOWS:

WHERE THE VETERAN IS STILL LIVING:

For those over age 65 but not housebound and not requiring regular aid and attendance:

For a veteran with no spouse or dependent
$1,021.00 per month

For a veteran with a spouse or one dependent
$1,337.00 per month

Housebound veterans:

For a housebound veteran with no spouse or dependent
$1,248.00 per month

For a housebound veteran with a spouse or dependent
$1,564.00 per month

For those in need of regular aid and attendance (A&A):

For an A&A veteran with no spouse or dependent
$1,703.00 per month

For an A&A veteran with a spouse or dependent
$2,019.00 per month

IF THE VETERAN IS DECEASED, THEN THE FOLLOWING LIST PROVIDES THE WIDOW'S/WIDOWER'S PENSION:

For those over age 65 but not housebound and not requiring regular aid and attendance:

For a widow(er) with no dependent
$684.00 per month

For a widow(er) with one dependent
$896.00 per month

Housebound widows/widowers:

For a housebound widow(er) with no dependent
$837.00 per month

For a housebound widow(er) with one dependent
$1,048.00 per month

For those in need of regular aid and attendance (A&A):

For an A&A widow(er) with no dependent
$1,094.00 per month

For an A&A veteran with one dependent
$1,306.00 per month

Under either list, add $174.00 per month for each additional dependent after the first dependent or spouse.

Also, you should know that if a widow or widower re-marries, then he or she can no longer qualify through his or her deceased veteran spouse. If a person divorces a veteran, that person is no longer eligible to qualify through the veteran he or she divorced.

Next let's look at a few examples of how this all fits together. For the purposes of these examples, we will assume that the asset requirement has been met. In our first example, we have a married couple living in assisted living. The veteran is in need of regular aid and attendance. The couple has a gross income of $48,000.00 per year.

Their unreimbursed health related expenses equal $60,000.00 per year. In this case, all of the income the couple has is paying for their care. In fact, they have a negative IVAP (remember IVAP is "Income for Veteran's Administration Purposes"):

$48,000.00 income

- $60,000.00 unreimbursed health care expenses

_____

-$12,000.00 IVAP

In this first example, the IVAP is negative as the couple's expenses are $12,000.00 more than their income each year. This means that in order to stay in assisted living, they will have to use their assets to pay for it, or hope a family member will help pay the bill. Since the couple has a negative IVAP, they would be entitled to the maximum Special Monthly Pension amount of $2,019.00 per month, or a bit more than $24,000.00 per year.

In the next example, the veteran is in an assisted living facility and in need of regular aid and attendance. The veteran's spouse lives at home. The family has a monthly income of $4,500.00. The unreimbursed health care expenses are $3,000.00 per month. The IVAP would be calculated as follows:

$4,500.00 income

- $3,000.00 unreimbursed health care expenses

_____

$1,500.00 IVAP

In this case, the maximum Special Monthly Pension amount is $2,019.00 per month. The VA will subtract the IVAP from the maximum pension amount to determine how much to pay.

$2,019.00 maximum Special Monthly Pension
- $1,500.00 IVAP

——————

$519.00 will be paid each month to the family

As you can see, if the family has income left over after paying the unreimbursed health care expenses, then this income (the IVAP) will be subtracted from the maximum Special Monthly Pension the veteran will receive. In fact, if the IVAP is greater than the Special Monthly Pension, then no pension will be paid, because the family does not pass the income limitation requirement.

Let's look at the previous example, but instead of the veteran being in assisted living, the veteran is housebound and has unreimbursed health related expenses of $900.00 per month.

$4,500.00 income
- $900.00 unreimbursed health care expenses

——————

$3,600.00 IVAP

Since the left over income ($3,600.00 of IVAP) is more than the maximum Special Monthly Pension for a housebound veteran with a spouse, which is $1,564.00, no pension will be paid.

Lastly, let's look at a widow who is in assisted living and needs regular aid and attendance. She has income of $2,500.00 per month from Social Security and her deceased husband's pension. Her unreimbursed health care expenses, including the assisted living facility's costs, are $3,500.00 per month.

$2,500.00 income

- $3,500.00 unreimbursed health care expenses

-$1,000.00 IVAP

Thus, this widow is $1,000.00 in the hole each month before applying for the Special Monthly Pension. The maximum pension for a widow in need of regular aid and attendance is $1,094.00. In this case, the widow will receive the full $1,094.00 per month, which will allow her to pay the balance of her assisted living bill each month.

In addition to educating clients about the Special Monthly Pension, elder law attorneys assist clients with planning strategies to help them obtain the Special Monthly Pension, while at the same time keeping an eye on the possible need for Medicaid in the future. Unlike Medicaid, which has a five year look-back period with regard to gifting (for more information, please read the Medicaid chapter of this book), currently the Special Monthly Pension benefit has no look-back period and no penalty period for gifts made prior to applying for the Special Monthly Pension.

However, before making any gifts to qualify for the Special Monthly Pension, you must have a second strategy in place. What if the veteran needs the gifted money back? What if the veteran ends up in a nursing home and needs to apply for Medicaid to pay the balance of the nursing home bill? Remember, the maximum Special Monthly Pension amount for a veteran with a spouse needing regular aid and attendance is $2,019.00 per month. While an extra

$2,019.00 per month may have been enough, along with the family income, to cover the household expenses and an assisted living bill, it probably won't be enough to pay the family expenses and a nursing home bill, which alone may run $5,000.00 to $9,000.00 per month depending upon where you live. Also, while the VA does not have a five year look-back period for gifts, Medicaid does, and Medicaid does not care that the VA failed to penalize you for the gift. This means Medicaid will penalize you for that same gift that the VA did not care about. In other words, if the veteran gives $75,000.00 to his or her child in order to qualify for the Special Monthly Pension, and then in three years, the veteran's health further declines, and the veteran goes to a nursing home and applies for Medicaid, that gift will prevent Medicaid from paying for the nursing home bill for approximately one year, because of the Medicaid imposed penalty on the gift! Will your child give the money back? What if your child dies, divorces, or gets sued?

Another thing to be careful of is people offering "free" VA planning, often using a strategy of gifting to family and purchasing annuities. Often both the gift and the annuity will cause problems if Medicaid is ever needed. We recommend that you never put a plan in place for the Special Monthly Pension without also putting a contingent plan in place for Medicaid.

The lesson here is do not let someone who is not knowledgeable about Medicaid help you with Special Monthly Pension planning. With a bad plan, the veteran could end up in worse shape than when he or she started. The gifted money might be gone, and Medicaid may impose a penalty because of the gift and another penalty because of the purchase of the non-qualifying annuity.

In recognition of the need for veterans and their families to get good advice, there are limited groups of people permitted to help veterans with Special Monthly Pension planning and applications. Those groups include Veteran Service Commissioners; recognized veterans service organizations, such as the VFW or American Legion; an agent accredited by the VA; and licensed attorneys accredited by the VA. Anyone else is not permitted to assist you and will likely cause you more harm than good. Further, even if a person can help you with the Special Monthly Pension, remember they need to also be knowledgeable about Medicaid so they do not unintentionally disqualify you for Medicaid down the road.

An elder law attorney accredited with the VA and knowledgeable concerning Medicaid can help a veteran devise a strategy that will help the veteran qualify for the Special Monthly Pension, while at the same time protect the veteran in case Medicaid is ever needed.

For more information, visit the website of
The Law Offices of Michael L. Brumbaugh Co., L.P.A. at:
http://www.brumbaughelderlaw.com.

CHAPTER 9

TRUSTS

Julieanne E. Steinbacher, CELA*
and
Adrianne J. Stahl, Esquire**

*Julieanne E. Steinbacher is a Certified Elder Law Attorney by
the National Elder Law Foundation and an Accredited Attorney
by the Veterans Administration

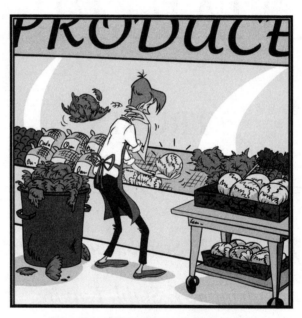

"THE DIFFERENCE BETWEEN
SALAD AND GARBAGE
IS A FEW DAYS!"

"LET OUR ADVANCE WORRYING BECOME ADVANCE THINKING AND PLANNING."

– Winston Churchill

§ 9.1.
INTRODUCTION TO TRUSTS

What is a "trust"? A trust is akin to a vehicle. "How?" you say. If you say "I have a trust" or "I want a trust," this is no more descriptive than you saying, "I drive a vehicle" or "I want a vehicle." Neither "trust" nor "vehicle" are very descriptive terms. What kind of trust is it that you have? What kind of trust is it that you want? Is the trust a revocable trust or an irrevocable trust? Is the trust an inter vivos (or living) trust or a testamentary trust? What kind of vehicle do you have? Is it a car, a truck, or an SUV? Is it a Chevy, a Ford, or a Toyota? What is the purpose of the trust? Is the purpose of the trust to protect assets from the costs of long-term care, to reduce federal estate taxes, or to protect against creditors? What is the purpose of the vehicle? Is the purpose of the vehicle to climb a mountain, to reduce gasoline costs, or to provide safe transportation?

There are as many different types and purposes of trusts as there are makes and models of vehicles. Often people visit a law office thinking that they need a trust, having notions of what a trust can and cannot accomplish, and thinking that all trusts are the same. On the contrary, a trust should be constructed to meet the individual goals of the person establishing the trust.

First, it must be understood what a trust is. A trust is a relationship between a settlor, a trustee, and the beneficiaries. A settlor (or donor or grantor) is the person who creates the trust and transfers property to the trust. The trustee is the person who administers the trust according to the terms of the trust. The beneficiary is the person or entity who benefits from, or will benefit from, the trust. There may be more than one settlor, trustee, and beneficiary of a trust. For instance, a husband and wife may create a trust (the husband and wife are the settlors/grantors/donors) for the benefit of their children (the beneficiaries) naming themselves as trustees of the trust. The trust document itself can be thought of as a written set of instructions (much like the owner's manual of a vehicle) from the settlor to the trustee for the benefit of the beneficiary. The trustee has a duty to follow the instructions in the trust and ensure that the goal or purpose of the trust is achieved.

§ 9.2.
TYPES OF TRUSTS

As mentioned earlier, there are as many types and purposes of trusts as there are vehicle makes and models. A trust may be created for almost any lawful purpose. A common reason for creating a trust is to provide for and protect someone. A property owner may want to convey property in trust to a minor, to an individual who lacks the skills necessary to manage property, to an individual who is prone to use property in an excessive or frivolous manner, or to an individual who is susceptible to influence from others. Trusts are not one-size-fits-all. Trusts must be customized to carry out the individual settlor's wishes.

Revocable v. Irrevocable Trusts

A revocable trust may be amended or terminated by the settlor during the settlor's life. Generally, an irrevocable trust may not be amended or terminated after it is created; however, states that have adopted some version of the Uniform Trust Code may allow an irrevocable trust to be modified or terminated upon the consent of the settlor and beneficiaries.

Testamentary v. Inter Vivos Trusts

A testamentary trust is created within a last will and testament and does not take effect until the death of the testator (the person who created the will). A testamentary trust does not avoid probate. A testamentary trust is revocable (can be changed by the testator/settlor) in the sense that a testator/settlor may execute a new will that revokes his previous will containing the testamentary trust. Upon the death of the testator/settlor, the testamentary trust takes effect and is irrevocable.

An inter vivos trust is created by the settlor during his life and becomes operative during the settlor's life. An inter vivos trust avoids probate. When the trust terminates, the property remaining in the trust is distributed according to the terms of the trust. The trust property does not pass pursuant to the settlor's last will and testament. An inter vivos trust may be either revocable or irrevocable.

As previously mentioned, a testamentary trust does not avoid probate, but an inter vivos trust does. Probate is the legal process wherein the estate of a decedent is administered. Generally, the probate process involves the personal representative collecting the decedent's assets, paying debts and taxes, and distributing property to beneficiaries or heirs. A decedent's probate estate consists of any property which does not pass upon death by another method. Examples of probate property include property owned solely by one person or by two or more people as tenants in common. Examples of nonprobate property include property owned as joint tenants with right of survivorship and contracts that provide for the payment of benefits upon death to a designated person, such as life insurance policies, retirement plans, annuities, and pay on death bank accounts.

Special Needs Trusts

A special needs or supplemental needs trust is a trust established for the purpose of providing benefits to and protecting the assets of a person who has a disability while allowing the person to receive governmental health and disability benefits, such as Supplemental Security Income (SSI), Medicaid, Social Security Disability (SSD),

Medicare, and Section 8 Housing. The assets in a special needs trust may be used to pay for the beneficiary's special and supplemental needs for which the government does not provide, which increases the beneficiary's quality of life.[54] Typically, a special needs trust prohibits a trustee from making distributions that provide the beneficiary with food or shelter because it is expected that public benefits, such as SSI, will provide for the beneficiary's food and shelter. Special needs trusts have a unique status within the world of long-term health care planning because assets may be transferred to a special needs trust to obtain immediate eligibility for Medicaid to pay for long-term care costs.[55]

§ 9.3.
TRUST V. OUTRIGHT GIFT:
THE FOUR D'S AND MORE

Trusts are effective tools for estate and long-term health care planning. A trust can be established to protect assets from the cost of nursing home care. Unfortunately, a nursing home stay or extended long-term care can destroy the financial security of a family, and the surviving spouse may suffer. Therefore, a husband and wife or a single individual may want to transfer assets to a trust to protect against the costs of long-term care.

The Four D's

When discussing the use of a trust to protect assets from the costs of long-term care, some people ask why they cannot just transfer their home and their other assets to their children rather than create a trust. The answer is not that their children are bad eggs. The answer is that life happens to all of us, and their children are no exception. Any one of us are vulnerable to the four D's – divorce, debt, disability, and death. No one likes to think that these things can happen to their children, but unfortunately they can, and do.

One or more of the children may get divorced, thereby putting the parents' assets at risk to equitable distribution in a child's divorce proceeding. Likewise, the children's creditors may collect against the parents' assets. Even if the children are currently debt free and able to meet their financial obligations, a child may be in a car accident for which the child is determined to be at fault. In this situation, the parents' assets may be at risk if the child is sued. Also, unfortunately, a child may become disabled at any time. For all of us, a disability is only an accident away. If a child becomes disabled, the child may not be able to take advantage of public benefits to assist him or her if the child owns the parents' assets. Furthermore, if a parent transfers his or her assets to a child, and the child dies, the parent's assets will pass through the child's estate to the child's beneficiaries, for instance, to the child's spouse.

The use of a trust can avoid the risks to the parents' assets associated with a child's divorce, debt, disability, and death. A trust may be written to include a spendthrift provision so that a beneficiary's creditors cannot reach the beneficiary's interest in the trust before the beneficiary actually receives a distribution from the trust. Additionally, a trust may be written to give the settlor the ability to change the beneficiaries of the trust. For instance, if the settlor's child becomes disabled, the settlor may want to remove the child as a beneficiary of the trust and instead name a special needs trust for the child's benefit. A special needs trust would provide benefits to and protect the assets of the child who has a disability while allowing the child to receive governmental health and disability benefits, such as Supplemental Security Income, Medicaid, Social Security Disability, Medicare, and Section 8 Housing. Furthermore, a trust may be written to provide for what happens to a beneficiary's share of the trust if the beneficiary predeceases the settlor or dies during the administration of the trust. For instance, the trust may provide that if the beneficiary dies, the beneficiary's interest in the trust passes to the beneficiary's children (as opposed to the beneficiary's spouse which may be the case when a trust is not used).

Medicaid Ineligibility Period

Beyond the risks of the four D's (divorce, debt, disability, and death), if parents gift assets outright to their children, the parents' assets will not be protected if their children or their children's spouses decide not to retain the assets for the parents' needs. When assets are transferred to a trust that protects from long-term care costs, the plan is that the trustee (or maybe a trust protector or a distribution committee – call it what you wish) is able to access the assets in the trust in the event the funds are needed. If parents gift assets outright to children, and the children spend the money, the money is no longer available if the parents' home needs a new roof, for instance, or if the parents want to go on a cruise.

Additionally, if the children spend the money gifted outright to them, there may be no money to pay for the parents' care during a Medicaid ineligibility period. Medicaid is a federal program funded by the federal and state governments, and the Medicaid rules vary from state to state. If an individual meets certain asset and income limitations, Medicaid will pay for nursing home care costs, and in some states, some in-home care costs. Generally, if a person requires nursing home care or in-home care and does not have any, or has insufficient long-term care insurance, he or she either has to pay the long-term care costs out of his or her own pocket or qualify for Medicaid to pay for them. A Medicaid penalty, or ineligibility period, is assessed for uncompensated transfers (gifts) made within the five years preceding the date of the Medicaid application (this is referred to as the "look-back period"). Transferring assets makes a person ineligible for Medicaid for one month for every $8,112.13 (this is the current penalty divisor in the Commonwealth of Pennsylvania; and this divisor varies from state to state) given away during what is known as the five-year look-back period (the period immediately before a person applies for Medicaid). The ineligibility period does not begin until the Medicaid application is filed and the applicant is determined to be eligible for Medicaid if it were not for the transfer(s).

If you transfer assets (either to another individual or to a trust), the transfers are subject to the Medicaid ineligibility period previously described. For example, if you transfer $100,000 today, a Medicaid ineligibility period of 12.3 months is created ($100,000 ÷ $8,112.13 = 12.3). If you would need long-term care within the next five years, the $100,000 would need to be reported to the Medicaid office at the time of the application. This 12.3 month ineligibility period begins on the date when the Medicaid application is filed and you are determined to be eligible for Medicaid if it were not for the transfer. This means that you would be required to privately pay for your in-home or nursing home care for at least 12.3 months. However, if you do not apply for Medicaid for at least five years from the date of the transfer, you would not have to disclose the transfer.

If parents gift assets outright to their children (as opposed to using a trust) and the children spend the money, there may be no money to pay for the parents' care during the Medicaid ineligibility period. In this situation, the nursing home may sue the children and the parents for payment. For more information on Medicaid benefits, please read the chapter of this book entitled *Medicaid.*

Income Taxes

On the beloved income tax side of things, another disadvantage of gifting assets outright to children is that when the children sell the property, the children will not receive a step-up in basis, which is a disadvantage to the children. The children's basis in the property will be the same as their parents' basis (the donors' basis).[56] On the contrary, if a grantor trust is used, the children's basis in the property will be the fair market value of the property on the date of the parents' death – the children will get a step-up or step-down in basis.[57]

There are other advantages of using a grantor trust for long-term care planning purposes. Grantor trusts do not need to be assigned an employer identification number (EIN).[58] Rather, these trusts may use the settlor's social security number. The major benefit of using a grantor trust is that it allows the settlor of the trust to remain in his or her individual marginal tax bracket. Another advantage of using a grantor trust is the settlor's ability to still be able to benefit from the Section 121 exclusion, which allows a taxpayer to exclude gain realized on the sale or exchange of real estate that was owned and used as the taxpayer's principal residence for at least two out of the five years preceding the date of the sale.[59]

A trust is a grantor trust for federal income tax purposes if the settlor of the trust retains certain powers or ownership benefits.[60] For instance, a trust is a grantor trust if the settlor of the trust has the power to add a beneficiary entitled to receive the principal or income of the trust.[61] Another instance of a grantor trust is one in which the settlor of the trust retains the right to the income from the property the settlor transfers to the trust.[62]

§ 9.4.
LONG-TERM CARE
PLANNING TRUSTS

"THROUGHOUT HISTORY WE HUMANS HAVE SOUGHT TO LIVE LONGER AND HEALTHIER LIVES. NOW THAT WE ARE ACHIEVING SOME SUCCESS, WE FIND WE CANNOT AFFORD TO GROW OLD."

– Anonymous

If an individual desires to create a trust to protect his or her assets from the cost of his or her long-term care, the trust must be created by the individual during his or her life (an inter vivos trust) and it must be irrevocable. Additionally, the individual cannot have access to the trust principal. Likewise, if the individual also desires to preserve the income of the trust from long-term care costs, the person cannot have access to the trust income. Many people are panicked by this. What if there is an emergency and they need the money in the trust?

When assets are transferred to a trust that protects from long-term care costs, the plan is that the trustee (or maybe a trust protector or a distribution committee) is able to access the assets in the trust in the event the trust funds are needed. Asset protection trusts can be written in such a way as to give a person whom the settlor trusts access to the trust income and principal.

§ 9.5.
TRUST FUNDING

A trust that is not funded is nothing more than a car with an empty tank of gas. A car exists without gasoline, but it is ineffective. An unfunded trust is equally ineffective. A trust can be funded during the settlor's life by changing ownership of existing assets or by purchasing new assets in the name of the trust. A trust can also be funded after the settlor's death by naming the trust as the beneficiary of life insurance policies, annuity contracts, or retirement plans. Additionally, in some circumstances, a trust may be funded with the assets of someone other than the settlor.

§ 9.6.
CONCLUSION

"ALL YOU NEED IS THE PLAN,
THE ROADMAP, AND THE COURAGE TO
PRESS ON TO YOUR DESTINATION."

– Earl Nightingale

Because we are living longer, our chances of needing long-term care are increasing. We now need to think about not only what happens if we die, but also what happens if we become ill and need long-term care. Estate planning attorneys answer the question "what happens if you die?" Elder law and long-term care planning attorneys answer the more difficult and important question "what happens if you do not die but become ill and need long-term care?" An elder law attorney does not simply prepare last will and testaments, trusts, and powers of attorney. An elder law attorney prepares a roadmap for you – a long-term health care plan to address your specific health care needs, financial situation, and individualized goals. Visit a trusted and experienced elder law attorney today for your own personalized long-term health care plan.

For more information, visit the website of
Steinbacher, Stahl, Goodall & Yurchak at:
http://www.paeldercounsel.com.

[54] 62 Pa. Stat. Ann. § 1414.

[55] 55 Pa. Code § 178.104(e)(2).

[56] I.R.C. § 1015(a).

[57] I.R.C. § 1014(a)(1); § 1014(b).

[58] U.S. Dep't of Treasury, IRS, 2010 *Instructions for Form 1041* at 12.

[59] I.R.C. § 121.

[60] U.S. Dep't of Treasury, IRS, 2010 *Instructions for Form 1041* at 11.

[61] See I.R.C. § 674.

[62] See I.R.C. § 677.

CHAPTER 10

END OF LIFE ISSUES

J. Randall Clinkscales, Esquire

Accredited Attorney by the Veterans Administration

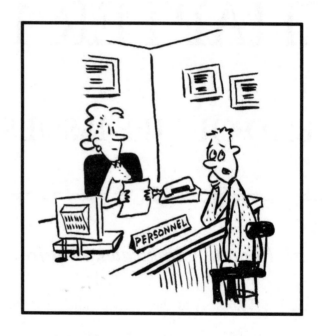

"I'M A DECISION-MAKER. WELL, I
THINK I AM. ON THE OTHER HAND,
I DON'T KNOW. AND THEN AGAIN..."

This was not the role he anticipated. His grandmother lived almost 600 miles away. When Grandmother had a heart attack in 2000, she was given only three to six months to live. In spite of the miles between them, he became her agent for financial and health care decisions.

For six years, he was a caregiver from afar. Then Grandmother's health failed, and, unhappily, he made a decision in 2006 to move Grandmother 600 miles away from her home to an assisted living facility near his home. It was a hard and difficult role for him, the decision-maker, and even more difficult, a decision not particularly welcomed by Grandmother.

Before the move, he and Grandmother had talked extensively. She knew that he was looking after her best interests. But it was still hard. She had lived in or around her hometown for all of her 92 years. As a result of the decision, she was going to move to a new state.

This was not the first decision he had been forced to make. Grandmother's driving skills had deteriorated with her failing eyesight. Lo and behold, Grandmother's car battery "suddenly" would not work one day. It just seemed like the car could not get fixed, and so Grandmother gave up driving.

Before the move, he made arrangements to oversee Grandmother's care in her own home. People began bringing lunch for Grandmother, but something about that rubbed Grandmother the wrong way, and she resisted the help. Grandmother summarily dismissed the caregivers. Eventually, two distant cousins began stopping by to check on Grandmother – and they reported to Grandson.

Grandmother's health began failing at a more precipitous rate. Twice, in six years, she went on hospice. So the decision in 2006 to move Grandmother out of her home and into assisted living was not Grandson's first exercise of authority, but it was his most difficult up to that time.

After the move in 2006, Grandmother actually did well in the assisted living facility though she suffered through a bout of depression that lasted a good six months. The depression was particularly hard on Grandson. He blamed himself. Eventually though, Grandmother made friends at the assisted living facility and became more social. Her health improved. During the next four years, there were "spells" – short bouts of illness that Grandmother recovered from, but never quite to the level she had been before the illness. Even though he had prepared a living will and health care power of attorney for her, the documents were nowhere to be found at the hospital when they might have been needed during a stay in the hospital. New ones were prepared.

He and Grandmother talked at length. She told him that she did not want any surgeries or CPR. They talked about a "Do Not Resuscitate," and she agreed that she wanted that.

Then, around Christmas of 2009, Grandmother fell ill. It was hard to figure out just what was wrong but she was not eating well.

As she was to be discharged from the hospital, the assisted living facility refused to take her back. Although he argued with the doctor, the hospital, and the assisted living facility, though he spoke harshly and threatened, it did no good. On December 31, 2009, Grandmother moved to a nursing home.

Grandmother was now 96. He had curtailed many of the medicines that she had been taking – at one time as many as 14. Many of them made her nauseous or exhausted. Without some of the medications, Grandmother was more alert and had more energy. But once the move to the nursing home was made, things were very different. She began refusing most nourishment – even chocolate shakes, her lifelong favorite confection. He kept getting reports about her condition from the nursing home and they were not good.

Each day he would see Grandmother. Sometimes he would paint her fingernails. There were only three options for the colors she preferred. He would hold her hands, remove the old polish and she would choose the new one. He would then apply the new, and she would look at her fingernails and brag to the nurses about his work. As he looked at Grandmother's hands, he recalled all of the times that she had bandaged his cuts and bruises, cooked meals for him and showed him her love.

One evening, he sat with Grandmother, holding her hands and polishing her nails. He was going to talk about her health and why she was not eating. He asked if she was not eating because perhaps she was sad or feeling poorly or just perhaps something else. This is what she said: "Honey, I know I am dying, and I am alright with that. The Lord has been good to me. But I just don't want you to worry about me anymore. It's okay for me to go now."

Three days later, after 56 days in the nursing home, Grandmother passed quietly. He was called that Thursday evening and arrived soon after her passing. He held her hands one last time, glad she had fresh polish on her nails.

As he prepared for Grandmother's funeral, he realized that she gave him and his family one of the most important gifts – the gift of knowing that she was ready to go and that she had accepted that. He realized that he had been able to participate in a process that gave her a higher quality of life and a dignity in death – and that the process had been a true partnership between him and his grandmother.

This is the story of my grandmother and me. I was fortunate that she and I could work together to experience her last days on her own terms.

The experience brought home to me the realities of end of life decisions. Have I done for my family, and for myself, what my grandmother did for me, and for herself? Have I prepared my affairs and my family for my disability or my death?

The landscape of dying has changed. While death can come suddenly, today death tends to come more slowly. Until the mid-1970s, most deaths were sudden: the three major causes of death were heart attacks, strokes, and accidents.

Today, the leading causes of death are gradual in nature. Examples of diseases that may lead to a gradual death include congestive heart failure, lung disease, diabetes, ALS (Lou Gehrig's Disease), Parkinson's, osteoporosis that results in falls, Alzheimer's, AIDS, and cancer.[63]

A trend toward more gradual death does not make end of life issues easier. In fact, it complicates them. The incidence of an accident; sudden illness; or even progressive, chronic illness can deprive us of the ability to participate in shaping end of life decisions.

There are a significant number of cases that discuss end of life decision making. One of the first important cases was the Karen Ann Quinlan case. In 1975, Quinlan, then 21 years of age, became unconscious after a party. Twice, she stopped breathing for fifteen minutes. Eventually, she slipped into a persistent vegetative state and was placed on a ventilator. After several months, her father sought to be her guardian. He requested the ventilator be discontinued, at his direction.

Initially, the New Jersey lower court denied the parents' request to discontinue the ventilator, and denied her father's request to be her guardian. The court went so far as to intimate that her father could be charged with murder if the ventilator was intentionally discontinued.

The case eventually landed in the New Jersey Supreme Court. That court found an individual has a right of privacy which could lead to the termination of the ventilator. If "the responsible attending physicians conclude that there is no reasonable possibility of Karen ever emerging from her present comatose condition to a cognitive, sapient state and that the life-support apparatus now being administered to Karen should be discontinued" and if a hospital ethic committee agreed, then the life support could be withdrawn; and that decision will be without any civil or criminal liability.[64]

The first "right to die" case before the U.S. Supreme Court was *Cruzan v. Director, Missouri Department of Health.*[65] In 1983, Nancy Cruzan was rendered incompetent as a result of an automobile accident. A gastrostomy feeding and hydration tube was surgically implanted in her body. Cruzan lapsed into a persistent vegetative state.[66] Her parents were appointed her co-guardians. They sought an order permitting the removal of their daughter's artificial feeding and hydration equipment after it became apparent that she had virtually no chance of recovering her cognitive faculties.

For the first time, the U.S. Supreme Court recognized that the U.S. Constitution grants a *competent* person a constitutionally protected right to refuse lifesaving hydration and nutrition.[67] However, it also found that the state (in this instance, Missouri) could establish procedural safeguards that had to be met before the wishes of an *incompetent* person, regarding withdrawal of treatment, would be honored. Missouri law required that proof of the wishes of an incompetent person must be established by clear and convincing evidence.[68]

Even though the Court ultimately found against the parents of Cruzan, the Supreme Court opened the door to a different result if her parents discovered ". . . new evidence regarding the patient's intent."[69]

Cruzan's parents seized on that language in the Supreme Court decision.[70] At a new trial, evidence was introduced regarding Nancy's wishes if she were in a vegetative state. Nancy had related to a co-worker that if she was ever a "vegetable," like Karen Ann Quinlan, she would not want to live.[71] The trial court granted Karen's parents' request for removal of the hydration and feeding tubes.[72] On Christmas Day, 1990, only a few days after the hydration and feeding tubes were removed, Nancy Cruzan died. The family's legal battle to remove the hydration and feeding tubes lasted eight years.[73]

Another difficult case of recent notoriety involved Theresa Schiavo. In 1990, Theresa, age 27, suffered a cardiac arrest with oxygen deprivation. As a result, she lapsed into a persistent vegetative state. Her husband, Michael, was appointed her guardian. After eight years, Michael filed a petition to discontinue artificial life support. The petition was opposed by Theresa's parents.[74] Theresa did not have a living will or any advance directive.[75] The only evidence of Theresa's wishes "were few and they were oral." The first court determined that even though there were only a few oral expressions, such expressions were sufficient to conclude Theresa would not want to live in a persistent vegetative state.[76]

Unfortunately, the finding was not the end of the battle. The husband and Theresa's parents continued to litigate, both at the state and federal level. The U.S. Congress became involved. The Florida Legislature even passed a law attempting to interfere with the litigation process. That attempt in the form of a law was eventually declared unconstitutional.[77]

What do we learn from this series of cases?

1. You have a constitutional right to refuse treatment if you are competent. It becomes much more complicated if you are not competent, unless you have adequately expressed your wishes.

2. You need to have effective documents that express your end of life wishes (perhaps a living will, "Declaration" in some states, and/or a power of attorney for health care, "Medical Proxy" in some states).

3. Express your wishes clearly (for instance, "If I am in a persistent vegetative state, I want the following services withheld: . . . feeding tube . . .").

4. Be sure that people know your wishes (someone knows you have a living will and/or health care power of attorney) and provide copies of your document or documents to your doctor and perhaps your hospital.

When reading this trilogy of cases, I realize how important it is to be sure that your whole family is well aware of what you want to happen – what is and what is not an acceptable quality of life to you. In my office, we call it "The Talk." We have our clients gather their family members together and have "The Talk" so that everyone is on the same page – their families understand my clients' desires about their end of life wishes. I do not want my clients to be the next important case that I read about in some law book. I cannot imagine going through what the Quinlan, Cruzan, and Schiavo families did at the most difficult of all times – the dying of a loved one.

What can you do now? Most important is to put your wishes and plans in place. How? Those wishes and your plans should be memorialized through a series of documents that should include a last will and testament and/or a trust (remember, a last will and testament will not be used until your death; a trust can be used by the family if you become incapacitated), a financial power of attorney, a health care power of attorney, and a living will. In some cases, when a person is terminally ill, or near the end of life, it may be appropriate to have the treating physician issue a "Do Not Resuscitate" order.

What issues do you want to address in these documents?

1. Who do you want to act for you? Clearly state who it is that you want to act or decide for you and what you want that person to decide. Name a backup to that person.

2. What do you deem is an acceptable or unacceptable quality of life? If certain conditions exist, what services are to be withheld? The unacceptable conditions could be defined to include terminally ill, in a persistent vegetative state, no brain activity, or unable to communicate in any fashion and no hope of recovering from that state. Then you may want to direct that you wish certain services are to be withheld: hydration, food, feeding tubes, blood transfusion, CPR, surgery, transplants, breathing apparatus, or insertion of artificial devices such as a pacemaker or defibrillator.

3. Do you want medical treatment decisions to comply with your religious beliefs? Do you want your health care agent or medical proxy to follow your religious beliefs? (As an example, some religions

do not believe in blood transfusions. That restriction can be placed in your planning documents.)

4. Do you want to be an organ donor? If so, to what extent? Most jurisdictions allow you to grant permission to your health care agent to determine to what extent your organs will or will not be donated.

5. If you become incapacitated, do you wish to live at home at any financial cost or will it be acceptable to place you in a nursing facility if that is the best alternative?

6. Can your financial and health care agent engage in financial planning so as to protect your assets from the cost of long-term care? An example would be allowing your family to protect assets for your "well spouse" so that he or she does not deplete your marital assets trying to care for you.

7. Do you want to use hospice care at the appropriate time? Hospice is a great program available through the Medicare system that provides care to you and even to your family, without cost.

8. If someone files a guardianship or conservatorship against you, who do you want the court to name as the guardian and conservator? You can name that person – someone you trust; someone who knows you and knows what you want.

9. Should your health care agent be authorized to obtain a "Do Not Resuscitate" order? A DNR is an order by a physician to not resuscitate a patient. Put that authority in your planning documents if that is what you want.

10. To what extent can pain management medication be used? What if the medication relieves your pain but could eventually hasten your death? If you want to authorize that course of treatment, put it in your planning documents.

I suggest that even at death, decisions will need to be made by someone. You can make them now in your planning documents.

1. What should happen to your remains? Are you to be buried or cremated?

2. Where do you want to be buried? Do you own a plot?

3. Do you want a funeral? You can prepay a funeral or set aside funds so that your funeral is not a financial burden for your family. You can even set out what type of music, scriptures, or whatever else you would like to have happen at your funeral (my grandmother did some of that, and it was a great help for me).

4. Do you want a memorial fund established in lieu of flowers? This is a wonderful way to continue to give, even after your death.

5. What memories do you want to leave your family? Consider making an ethical will or a family love letter that tells your family about what was important to you during your lifetime and what you hope they remember about your life. Include a history of the family. It is an invaluable gift.

We are all going to die. While we cannot dictate every term of our death, we can certainly prepare for it in advance. Preparation allows us to die, as best we can, on our own terms and in accordance with our own wishes. We can die in such a way that our family can feel at peace that whatever wishes we had were carried out in the best manner that the circumstances would allow.

For more information, visit the website of
Clinkscales Elder Law Practice, P.A. at:
http://clinkscaleslaw.com.

[63] Kiernan, Steven P., *Last Rights: Rescuing the End of Life from the Medical System* 7-8 (2007).

[64] *In the Matter of Karen Quinlan*, 70 N.J. 10, 24, 355 A.2d 647, 671 (1976).

[65] *Cruzan v. Director, Missouri Department of Health*, 497 U.S. 261, 110 S. Ct. 2841 (1990).

[66] *Id.* at 265-66.

[67] *Id.* at 279.

[68] *Id.* at 280.

[69] *Id.* at 283.

[70] Used with permission from Colby, William H., *Long Goodbye: The Deaths of Nancy Cruzan* 322 (2002).

[71] *Id.* at ch. 37.

[72] *Id.* at 361.

[73] *Id.* at 386.

[74] *In re Guardianship of Theresa Marie Schiavo v. Michael Schiavo*, 780 So. 2d 176, 177 (Fla. Dist. Ct. of App. Second District) (2001) (commonly referred to as Schiavo I).

[75] *Id.* at 178.

[76] *Id.* at 180.

[77] *Bush v. Schiavo*, 885 So. 2d 321 (Fla. 2004).

CHAPTER 11

PITFALLS, PROBLEMS, AND THINGS TO LOOK OUT FOR WHEN CONSIDERING LONG-TERM CARE PLANNING

Michael L. Brumbaugh

Accredited Attorney by the Veterans Administration

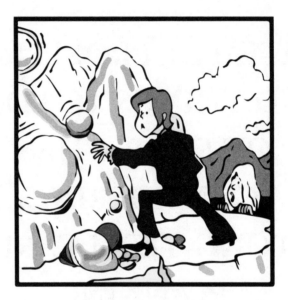

*"NEVER MIND THOSE!
KEEP YOUR EYE ON THE GOAL!"*

§ 11.1.
INTRODUCTION

In this chapter, we will consider some of the more common problems we see people encounter when they fail to plan or try to plan and do so poorly. Often, these two areas overlap, and it can be difficult at times to determine whether someone failed to plan or planned poorly. However, the outcome is generally the same and typically results in an unnecessary spend down of assets and a failure to protect the options and independence of the declining senior. Like many of the topics in this book, this chapter could be a book in and of itself. Thus, this chapter only hits some of the many things that could be covered under this topic.

§ 11.2.
JOINT AND SURVIVOR ACCOUNTS

All too often we see a parent add a child's name to bank accounts. Often the parent does this as a matter of convenience so the child can then access the accounts on behalf of the parent. Frequently, the parent adds the child to accounts in order to keep the accounts out of probate. Sometimes the parent adds a child to accounts under the mistaken belief that the accounts are then protected from Medicaid and nursing homes. Generally, the parent does not know the potential problems created by adding the child to the accounts.

When a child's name is added to an account that child becomes an owner along with the parent. The child can draw out the entire account balance and use the money for himself. Further, if the child gets divorced, the account might be considered by the divorce court as an asset of the child's to be divided in the divorce proceedings. Even if the court ultimately decides that the spouse of the child is not entitled to any of the account, the account might be tied up in expensive litigation for a long period of time.

Another pitfall that can result where a parent has added a child to the parent's account occurs if the child gets sued. If that happens, the parent's account might be attached to pay for the child's debts and judgments since the child is a co-owner on the account. Are you certain your child will never be in a car accident where he is at fault? Car accident claims often exceed the value of the insurance, and if that happens, the plaintiff can go after other assets owned by the driver – such as your account!

Another thing most people don't realize when they put a child on an account is that the ownership is usually joint with rights of survivorship. This means that when the parent dies, the account does not pass through the parent's Will, but instead the surviving child automatically owns the account. If there is only one child, this might not be a big deal. However, if a parent has multiple children and the parent's Will leaves the parent's assets equally to all of the children, then the parent's intention will not be followed insofar as the co-owned accounts legally go to just one child – the child who was on the account.

Furthermore, adding a child to an account does not help with regard to Medicaid and nursing home planning. The entire account balance will still be considered by Medicaid as being owned by the parent except to the extent that the child can prove she actually contributed some of her own money to the account.

§ 11.3.
NO ESTATE PLAN/CAN'T FIND THE ESTATE PLAN/BAD ESTATE PLANS

There are many reasons a person may not plan his estate. Some of those reasons are covered in the chapter of this book on Myths and Misunderstandings (such as the mistaken belief no estate plan is needed). Sometimes people are superstitious and truly believe that estate planning is bad luck! Others believe there will always be time to plan their estate and that they will get to it later or when the time is right.

For the person that doesn't know he needs an estate plan, a little bit of education can solve this mistaken belief. One way to educate the person is to give him a copy of this book!

For those individuals who believe there is always time to plan, sometimes a gentle nudge is needed to let them know that if they wait too long, they may not be able to plan their estate at all. They might be jeopardizing their independence and unnecessarily risking their assets, and they may cause their family members unnecessary work and heartache. An example of this occurrence is where a guardianship is needed due to a lack of an estate plan.

As to those individuals who are superstitious, we often must educate them, letting them know the importance of planning and being patient with them. Even if only the most basic estate plan is put in place, many pitfalls can be avoided. For example, most guardianships can be avoided just by executing a power of attorney. Further, if an elder law attorney helps create the estate plan, there will be tools in the estate plan permitting Medicaid planning if it is ever needed.

Even worse (or at least sadder) than having no estate plan is the person who puts an estate plan in place, then "hides" the documents so well that they cannot be found when needed. Sometimes the documents truly are hidden, and even though the family knows an estate plan was created, the documents can't be found. Generally, if the documents can't be found, the effect is the same as if no estate plan had ever been created. Sometimes the documents aren't hidden on purpose, but the family doesn't know there is an estate plan or where to find the documents. If you have an estate plan, make sure your family (at least those persons named as decision makers in the documents) knows you have one and knows where to find the original documents.

You may wonder how an estate plan can be bad. Estate plans can become bad for a number of reasons. One way is where an estate plan is created and put away and never looked at again. Often such plans have people named as decision makers who are no longer appropriate and sometimes aren't even alive! The plans might leave out children born after their creation, or the plans might not provide for grandchildren. The lesson here is you need to pull out your estate plan every couple of years and see if it still makes sense.

Another problem is harder for people to see on their own and will likely require that an elder law attorney review the estate plan. Many times, estate plans are created by attorneys who do not practice elder law. Such estate plans generally are fine for getting assets to the right people on death; or if a revocable trust is used, the trust generally is a fine tool for avoiding probate. However, the documents usually have no language in them for Medicaid and nursing home planning. In fact, we often see documents that actually restrict Medicaid planning. An example of this is a financial power of attorney that prevents or limits gifts. An often-used strategy in preserving assets in Medicaid planning is to make strategic transfers to a spouse (even though to a spouse, this is still a gift) or other family members. Such a strategy might be prevented by restrictive language in the power of attorney or a power of attorney that has no Medicaid planning language.

§ 11.4.
A FAILURE TO REALIZE THAT GIFTS ARE BEING MADE

The Medicaid rules take a very harsh position on gifts and look back five years to determine if gifts (called "improper transfers" by Medicaid) have occurred. In addition to many people not even knowing there are problems with gifting, even more people don't know what might be considered a gift.

Depending on the part of the country you live in, the following may be considered gifts that cause a transfer penalty to be imposed by Medicaid: Christmas gifts to your children and grandchildren, wedding gifts, graduation gifts, paying tuition for a child or grand-child, giving to charities, giving to your church, etc. We are not saying you should stop making such gifts, but we do encourage you to find out the possible effects such gifts might have on you if you ever need Medicaid so that you don't have any nasty surprises. Gifts are often fine if done as part of a well thought out plan created with the assistance of an elder law attorney.

Adding a child's name to real estate causes a gift. Selling an asset for less than it is worth causes a gift equal to the amount Medicaid says you undersold the property.

Another area where unsuspecting gifts can occur can be called the "incomplete gift." We have seen parents "give" their children vehicles and even real estate, and the "gifts" were made more than five years prior to the parent needing Medicaid. However, since the title was never transferred, the gifts were not complete as far as Medicaid is concerned. We've seen parents actually deed their real estate to their children, but then require their children to sign a promissory note for the property in which the parents state they never intended the children to pay. So, while the transfer of the real estate was a completed gift, the promissory note became a new asset of the parents, and as far as Medicaid is concerned, however much is owed on the promissory note, is treated the same as cash in the pocket of the parents.

§ 11.5.
MAKING GIFTS WITHOUT REGARD TO PENALTY PERIODS

When a gift is made, it will cause a penalty period to be imposed by Medicaid if the gift was made within five years of needing Medicaid. It is not unusual for parents to give large sums to their children, such as $13,000.00 per year, as the parents age. However, if nursing home care and Medicaid are needed, those gifts can cause serious penalties under Medicaid's rules such that Medicaid will not pay for care during the penalty period. Often, gifting can still be done, but it should be done with a plan put in place first. You must have a plan that covers the possibility that Medicaid will be needed within five years of the gift being made. Not having a plan is like jumping out of an airplane without a parachute.

§ 11.6.
IGNORING TAX CONSEQUENCES

Another problem we see again and again when people try to do their own Medicaid planning is ignoring the effect gifts have on taxes. When a person gifts an asset, the tax basis transfers to the person who receives the gift. The best way to demonstrate this is with an example. Let's say Mom and Dad bought their home in 1950 for $20,000.00. Now, their home is worth $120,000.00. Mom and Dad pass away owning the house, and their executor sells the house for $120,000.00. No capital gains tax will be owed under the current tax code because of how the IRS treats assets that pass to people upon death.

However, if the parents gift their home to their children, an entirely different tax result occurs. Let's assume that the children sell the house for $120,000.00. If we forget about any expenses related to the sale for the sake of simplicity, the IRS will say that capital gains taxes are owed on the $100,000.00 profit ($120,000.00 sale price less the $20,000.00 Mom and Dad paid for the house). At a 15% capital gains tax rate, the taxes owed because Mom and Dad gifted the property before death would be $15,000.00. As you can see, the IRS treats the taxes on assets sold, after they have been gifted, much differently than those assets that transfer because of someone passing away.

Finally, let's consider one more tax trap. Mom and Dad gift their home to their children and continue to live in the house. Six years after making the gift, Mom and Dad move out of the house to independent living, and the house is sold for $120,000.00. Again, capital gains tax would be owed on the $100,000.00 profit. This tax would not have been owed if Mom and Dad had sold the property while it was in their names as the IRS has a capital gains exclusion for the sale of your personal home.

§ 11.7.
BELIEVING MEDICAID OR THE NURSING HOME WILL ASSIST YOU WITH MEDICAID PLANNING

It is not the job of the Medicaid agency or the nursing home to tell you how to use Medicaid's rules to help you preserve assets. The Medicaid agency basically processes your application and tells you whether you are approved for Medicaid. Even if the Medicaid agent sees ways you can preserve assets, she is unlikely to tell you.

Nursing homes receive more pay for people paying out of their own pocket than they do for those on Medicaid. Further, the person at the nursing home that assists the nursing home's clients in applying for Medicaid is not trained to know the strategies available to preserve assets. Her job for the nursing home is to assist those clients in applying for Medicaid who have spent down their assets by paying their money to the nursing home. Her job does not include telling you all the strategies to keep you from having to pay your money to the nursing home. In fact, she might get in trouble with her employer, the nursing home, if she starts telling you such strategies, assuming she even correctly knows any.

§ 11.8.
FAMILY CONFLICTS

Things go much smoother with a plan. There still might be bumps but if you have a roadmap or plan to guide you, the journey will go easier than without a plan. You owe it to yourself and your family to give them guidance as to what you desire and who you want in charge when life throws challenges at you.

No one knows better than you about the strengths and weaknesses in your family. You might love all your children equally, but there may be one or more children that you would never want to be in charge of your money. You might also have someone in your family that is more likely to stir up trouble than to make things go smoother. You can make life easier for everyone with a well thought out estate plan that takes such matters into consideration.

Conflicts can also arise when family members disagree on the condition of a parent. It is fairly common for children that live far away from a parent not to realize how much the parent's health has declined, especially when dementia is involved. The child that lives far away may not interact with the parent often enough to see the decline. Plus, many persons who have dementia are able to mask its symptoms so long as they are in familiar surroundings. When a child that lives close to the parent informs the other child that Mom or Dad is starting to have serious memory impairment issues, the child that lives far away may just not see those issues. Moreover, sometimes the child that doesn't interact with Mom or Dad as much may have feelings of guilt about not being more involved, and this increases the odds that child will be in denial. There is no easy solution to such problems. However, having an estate plan in place beforehand with plans about what the parent wants and who is in charge will go a long way. Further, regular conversation among family members before the situation becomes a crisis can be very beneficial so that there is less chance a child is surprised by the parent's decline in health.

§ 11.9.
CONCLUSION

While pitfalls and problems are a part of life, many of the problems and pitfalls people face concerning planning for later life can be avoided if they sit down with an elder law attorney and discuss their fears, wishes, and goals and create a comprehensive estate plan.

For more information, visit the website of
The Law Offices of Michael L. Brumbaugh Co., L.P.A. at:
http://www.brumbaughelderlaw.com.

AFTERWORD

I know from personal experience how difficult it is to deal with the challenges presented when a loved one is no longer able to care for him or herself. In my case it was my mother who had gotten up in years and was no longer able to function independently. It's tough because we want to remember our parents (and our grandparents too) as the vital and energized people that we looked to for guidance and direction while we ourselves were growing up.

However, with the passing years, the roles more often than not get reversed, and now it is we as adults who are called on to care for and make decisions for our elderly loved ones. The result is that it feels as if the weight of the world is now on our shoulders as we deal with the guilt and pressure of making a vitally important caregiving decision. This decision can't be taken lightly, and because of this we, as responsible children and grandchildren (sometimes even as a husband or a wife), seek to discover as much information as possible to insure that we make the absolute best caregiving choice possible.

This is what led me to create *The Choices for Care Program* on DVD (more information and sample footage available at www. ChoicesforCare.com/index.php?aff=JS) and also become finely tuned to any other valuable resources that can aide in your discovery process. I've found such a resource within the pages you just read courtesy of one of our nation's leading elder law attorneys, Julie Steinbacher. She has meticulously selected a group of her fellow elder law attorneys for their talent, expertise, and experience in the individual subject matter that each has been asked to write about in this book.

Speaking of this publication, as I sit here and write this, I have no idea what the investment has been for you to obtain a copy. However, from the value of the information you have just read, I can say without hesitation that a price of at least $100.00 would have been my recommendation. Even at this figure, it would still wind up being one of the best bargains you will get this year! Why? Because dollar-for-dollar you cannot put a price tag on the wisdom and counsel you've received within this book and the comfort and confidence you've gotten after pouring through these pages.

As someone who has come to appreciate the dedication those in the elder law profession bring to the table every day of their professional lives, I'm confident you are now prepared to embark on a journey that will make you all the more richer for coming into contact with the outstanding men and women you have met in this book.

Chip Kessler
Johnson City, TN
Creator, Developer, & Producer of
The Choices for Care Program